Don't Mess with My Mojo

Dear Lisa
Wishing you happy Mojo moments!
From Liesa with an "e"
X

Don't Mess with My Mojo

A Handbook for Sparking a Sassy Morning

LIESA OTTO

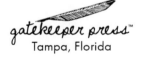
Tampa, Florida

The views and opinions expressed in this book are solely those of the author and do not reflect the views or opinions of Gatekeeper Press. Gatekeeper Press is not to be held responsible for and expressly disclaims responsibility for the content herein.

DON'T MESS WITH MY MOJO:
A Handbook for Sparking a Sassy Morning

Published by Gatekeeper Press
7853 Gunn Hwy., Suite 209
Tampa, FL 33626
www.GatekeeperPress.com

Copyright © 2024 by Liesa Otto

All rights reserved. Neither this book, nor any parts within it may be sold or reproduced in any form or by any electronic or mechanical means, including information storage and retrieval systems, without permission in writing from the author. The only exception is by a reviewer, who may quote short excerpts in a review.

Library of Congress Control Number: 2023933626

ISBN (paperback): 9781662931314

To my tribe of worldwide wonder women,
your sass brings moments of joy to every occasion.

In memory of my treasured mum and dear dad,
who started my story.

*Mojo is embracing shameless self-love.
It is the essence and energy of joy.
And it's within each of us.*

Contents

Let's Begin 11
How to Use This Book 20

Mind

The Power of the FAFF: 23
The Fabulous Art of Feeling Fulfilled

Juicy Self-Journaling: 32
Release Your Real Self and Lose Your Mind

Groom Your Goal-tention: 40
Ignite Your Intention into Action

Body

Manifest a Move: 51
Body Language for Moving Vividly

The Naked Smoothie: 66
Strip It Down and Suck It Up

Soak Your Inner Self: 78
Sassy Sips for Perfect Hydration

Heart

Glow with Gratitude: 89
Awaken Your Awe and Count Your Blessings

Shameless Self-Love: 97
Brush Up Your Senses One Stroke at a Time

Spirit

Ms. Meditation Maven: 107
Breathe In and Let It Flow

"Scentual" Awareness: 116
Get in the Mood in a Whiff

Meltdowns, Mindset, and Mojo 124
Living MoJOYfully 126

Let's Begin

You've landed:
Right here, right now, you're in the right place. Just breathe.
Sink into yourself—surrender to discovery.
Dare to imagine—join the joyride. Greet
the Goddess within. Invite her
to start and stay in her
day with presence,
sass, and
joy.

Before my mornings became manageable, they were mostly messy. Waking up was easy enough; I'm an efficient getter-upper most days. However, from the time my feet hit the floor until my official workday started, I was Queen Faffalot. My body and brain were rarely in sync, and I dithered, flapped, and fretted my way through the morning, achieving absolutely not a lot. I was the consummate faffer! For those of you who aren't up on your British slang, a faffer is someone who wastes time or procrastinates. You could say that "faff" stands for the Frustrating Art of Fussing and Flapping (and yes, sweet reader, I will take you on a wild journey through this fascinating phenomenon in the upcoming chapter).

    I perfected the skill of faffing while living in the tropics of Papua New Guinea, where I taught grade school. In my professional life, I was Little Ms. Mighty, but at home, I would morph into Big Mismanagement—especially during the first hours of my day. Morning would appear with her golden, smiling island face, and I would greet her, green with envy and scowling in the corner like a petulant child.

My mornings were anything but fabulous. They always started similarly: stumbling down to the kitchen to get my coffee fix had priority over absolutely *everything*—which had me racing back up two flights of stairs to the bathroom with little notice. (What was I, five years old?)

Mornings were peppered with indecision, procrastination, and unsuccessful attempts to multitask. I would quickly skim emails as I simultaneously hustled for an outfit to wear and pondered over the evening's dinner options, all while my sweet little brain took a quick guilt trip to the Land of Unsettling Thoughts. I'd make lunches I forgot to pack and promises I failed to keep. Random lists were scribbled on rogue scraps of paper, only to be misplaced. I became so hot and bothered that the other humans in my house became the unsuspecting victims of my snarkiest wit. I was one storm away from a Coral Sea shipwreck!

I was discouraged and irritated when I clambered into my car to drive to work each day; my stomach was already rumbling. Wolfing down a granola bar is less than ideal, and I was anxiously churning over the day's potential problems. The only routine I managed to stick with was undertaking the daily safety check before I departed my compound. I couldn't forget that this beautiful island was affectionately nicknamed the Land of Unexpected. Doors locked, my mobile phone discreetly positioned in my bra, personal radio turned on. Check, check, check! The blacked-out car windows drew me deeper into my opaque cocoon, while the transparent strip of glass in front of me promised clarity, at least for a little while.

Nailing the art of self-sabotage was easy, but self-care? It felt like trying to get a teenager out of bed on a weekend. An ongoing series of mayhem and mishaps. My faffing was more "Groundhog Day" than I'd ever signed up for.

Was this how I wanted my days to unfold forever more? *Something needed to change.*

Taking full responsibility for my mishandled mornings, I embraced the role of my own daring experiment, diving headfirst into the process of self-discovery. Listening closely to my inner voice, I faced head-on the obstacles that had held me back for far too long. Shifting my mindset to one of self-love, I began an eye-opening and transformative journey of self-care. By the time the southeast monsoon season ended, I had reinvented and reprioritized my mornings, finally allowing me to pay attention to some of my unmet needs.

Completing bathroom routines *first thing* meant my basic physical needs were met from the get-go. From there, eating a nutritious breakfast ensured I was fueled for the day ahead, and learning to sit with my thoughts—instead of loudly trying to untangle them with my loved ones—granted me the headspace and sanity to avoid a potential combat zone.

Some of these habits seemed too simple. Yet, they were exactly what I craved, and the satisfaction I got from sorting out these small tasks injected little bursts of happiness into my day. Something amazing started happening. I was unearthing my mojo.

Most dictionaries will tell you that 'mojo' is all about personal power and a touch of magic. I'm completely smitten with that idea! It's like uncovering the sweet spot where your superpowers and individual mystique lovingly collide. Ever since my empowering discovery, I've become a seeker of mojo—what I see as the essence and energy of joy.

My journey to understanding mojo has been more of a backpacking adventure than a five-star resort experience. On this trek, I have embraced the unexpected; I've explored new paths and met new ideas along the way. There were bumps in the road, check-backs, and deep ravines. But when I found myself rounding a corner to witness the most beautiful waterfall, where I could dip my tired toes into the cool, sparkling water, I finally understood what mojo was all about.

As a Mojo-ologist, I'm on a lifelong mission to beat procrastination, invite that sweet flow state, and sprinkle special moments into my daily mix. Over the years, I've delved into nutrition, exercise, wellness, and self-improvement, seeking the perfect tools for my mojo-loving spirit. We're on this journey together, my clients and I. 'Mojo' isn't just a word; it's become a sassy shorthand for Moments of Joyful Occasion.

Each morning, as we climb out of bed to face the day, we enter a world of endless possibilities. Taking a cue from the creative guru Julia Cameron, the mastermind behind *The Listening Path* and *The Artist's Way*, we stumble upon a golden 45-minute window right after waking up. It's our little escape from the clutches of our ego's defenses. It's a time to connect with our true selves, drop the facades, and embrace authenticity. In these early moments, mojo is at its freshest and most vibrant.

Our morning sets the scene for how our thoughts and actions take shape, how productive and calm the day will be, and even how we approach difficult situations that might arise. You know the feeling if you've ever opened a tough email first thing in the morning. It somehow seems worse before 7:00 a.m. and can make you reactive all day. When the outer world collides with our beautiful and messy inner world—BOOM! Would you like a slice of the apocalypse with your coffee? On the other hand, fill your mind with something positive so that throughout your day, you will attract more of the same—and you will be able to better cope with that prickly email.

Imagine a morning self-care practice that feels real to you and where you start choosing yourself. Your needs are met head-on, from the get-go, and become part of your everyday life. How amazing would that be? Well, this doesn't need to be a fantasy! I've had clients who have experienced remarkable changes in their energy levels and overall happiness since participating in group fitness classes within the first few hours after waking.

Others have declared that since establishing a new self-love routine and making themselves a priority, there were fewer family feuds and raised voices before school. They felt more at peace, more connected to themselves and those around them. If you set up your morning lovingly, the rest of the day will energetically follow with ease.

Let's look at the difference between routine and ritual. Routines like brushing your teeth or making your bed focus on an outcome and aren't necessarily motivating or joy-inducing activities. We just get the job done without too much thought. Conversely, a ritual is established once a routine becomes *intentional* because the actions bring meaning, learning, or joy into our life—such as the rituals in this book! Magic happens when that intentional ritual manifests into daily practice. Creative and teacher Mary Thoma, whose practice includes healing and ritual, describes this as "a combination of consistent and evolving devotional activities that help ease you in the direction of remembering and connecting to your True Self." Each ritual can become its own practice, as can the combinations of rituals that contribute to your unique Morning Practice.

Three "un-qualities" killed my mojo during my early days in Papua New Guinea: procrastination, a shortage of self-prioritization, and constantly being in an early-morning productivity deficit. I realize that when these life-sucking forces dominate my days, I scramble to make sense of anything. Maybe you know that empty, overwhelming—or underwhelming—feeling in the pit of your stomach. It might feel like that sweet little spark that kept you ignited has gone out.

Self-care can be hard to figure out and may feel arduous, like you have to do it all and make it #justperfect. But let me pop that overinflated balloon and offer a more sustainable, authentic approach. Research shows that when we make things enjoyable, we persist for longer and achieve more. So, why not infuse some excitement into self-care?

Before we dive into what self-care is, firstly, let's clear the buzz about what it isn't. Self-care is not an indulgence or being selfish. Nor is it something we force ourselves to do because we think we should. It's not something we reach for when we're at the end of our rope, and it's definitely not the platitudes and empty promises of the multimillion-dollar self-care industry. When you wholeheartedly meet your mental, emotional, and physical needs daily, and this fills you up, igniting the brightest parts within you—this is self-care at its best. It's an empowering and deliberate commitment to your well-being. That's what mojo is all about, and let me tell you, it feels effing fabulous!

"*Well, then,*" you may ask, "*how do I successfully mastermind my self-care practice?*"

With a bit of sass and self-love, sweet reader.

A Handbook for Sparking a Sassy Morning

I had moved from Papua New Guinea to Indonesia when two unexpected back-to-back events shattered my mojo, and it seemed like the universe had become the biggest asshole ever. After a series of surgeries to try to preserve my painfully arthritic hip joints, I was recovering in a hospital in Singapore when I learned that my father was terminally ill. This news prompted me to leave my life and family in Indonesia and fly to New Zealand to be with him.

Hobbling through my days on crutches, I went into full caretaker mode. I became laser-focused on the minutia, scheduling medications and bucket lists, counting pills and days, and cajoling everyone's frayed nerves while nervously waiting for a ball to drop. As my emotional bandwidth started to resemble white noise, I knew I needed to rally my self-care in the wake of my obligations.

As I reminisced about my time on the islands, I couldn't help but recall the small changes I made to my daily routines. Giving myself grace once more, I started to listen to my inner voice from a place of self-love. "Take a daily walk," my body gently suggested, while my mind urged me to express my thoughts, grief, and hopes. My heart reminded me to appreciate the many blessings in my life, and my spirit nudged me to find solace in moments of quiet stillness. Upon returning to Jakarta after a few months, with healed hips and a sense of guidance and grounding, my curiosity about rituals and self-care was ignited even further. As I fine-tuned my daily routine while taking care of my dad, I discovered unexpected moments of hope and joy. It was then I realized that joy and sorrow could coexist harmoniously. I wanted to celebrate life's little moments, no matter the circumstances. Embracing those fleeting joys became my way of cherishing the beauty of each day.

So, I returned to school and immersed myself in studying. I questioned, I listened, and I delved into the creation and testing of my hypotheses. Then, I pressed 'repeat.' It was through this process that I discovered the transformative power of repairing and integrating the four holistic elements—the mind, body, heart, and spirit—into my self-care practice. These cornerstones of well-being became my guide, and I finally found the medicine I needed. The result? A significant shift in my joy factor.

This book came to life through a blend of experimentation, careful curation, and a genuine passion. I extensively researched and drew from my personal journey to curate ten beautiful morning rituals that seamlessly resonate with the mind, body, heart, and spirit. These aren't your usual self-help tasks—they're more like little boosts of inspiration and confidence that give your mornings that extra kick of energy and zest.

Imagine taking a conventional activity (like journaling) and adding a new twist, or embracing an unconventional activity (such as faffing) and, from this, designing something unique. Each up-leveled ritual is infused with a bit of sass, and my daily practice now pops with curiosity, freshness, and fun.

The rituals are interconnected; they complement one another and, separately or combined, will create your morning practice. For example, when we meditate, we can access our more conscious self, which can shift our intentions. Journaling after meditating might feel particularly productive, as might practicing gratitude.

I love these juicy words by Martha Beck, author of *The Way of Integrity*: "When you experience unity of intention, fascination, and purpose, you live like a bloodhound on a scent, joyfully doing what feels truest in each moment." This description makes me want to grab every colored pen I own and wildly color my day.

If your mojo is missing—whether it has been taken away or if you just haven't found it yet—this handbook will help you. My hope, sweet reader, is that you can be curious and adopt one or more of these rituals to lightly tether your mornings, so there are fewer 'F-bombs' (frustration, fussing, and flapping) and way more MOJO!

How to Use this Book

Your engagement and effort truly make a difference. With a little commitment, you can kick-start a new habit. Stick with it, and you'll see intentional change unfolding, guiding you on a journey that feels just like your own. For the most part, these rituals don't require much time. However, things can sometimes get in the way. When the unexpected calamity arises, like a cheetah loose in the living room or waking up to a queasy stomach after far too much broccoli (this happened to me, I'm a little embarrassed to say), it's enough to let it be. Regroup and rest—and then try again tomorrow.

As you build ritual into your morning, there may be times when you need to scale down your practice for a moment. One or some of the rituals all the time, all the rituals some of the time, or whatever-ritual-I-can-manage-today-at-any-time, is an acceptable way of doing things. Just show up and do what you can.

To help you successfully implement your morning practice, I suggest you approach your chosen rituals with four critical factors in mind. These have greatly helped me stay motivated and consistent:

1. **Block and prioritize your time.**
2. **Celebrate each ritual and make it sacred.**
3. **Review your ritual/s regularly.**
4. **Go gently into your practice.**

This isn't a sprint. It's more like a slow and steady race that we can begin together. Take out your version of a sparkly gel pen, sweet reader, and let's start exploring your morning story.

Mind

THE POWER OF THE FAFF
The Fabulous Art of Feeling Fulfilled

Today's To-'Done' List

- ☑ Make the magnanimous "to-do" list
- ☑ Let the mind wander
- ☑ (Joyfully) stroll through the house naked as a jaybird
- ☑ Reorganize spatulas
- ☑ Rearrange fridge magnets
- ☑ Eat (multi-grain) Cheerios from the box while gazing out the dirty windows
- ☑ Search for the Windex (finally find it)
- ☑ Clean two dirty windows with gusto (while listening to Natasha Bedingfield's 'Unwritten.')
- ☑ Lose interest
- ☑ Feel overly underwhelmed and unproductively over it
- ☑ Get dressed
- ☑ Check off nothing on the magnanimous "to-do" list

Shoulders back, chest out, I'm poised on a Swiss Ball at my immaculate work desk, a steaming espresso waiting expectantly, my laptop open with anticipation. Soft and eager finger pads beckon toward the warm, hard keys. Oh, the blessed report; I need to put you to bed *right now!* But wait—the tangled mess of electronic cords beneath the chair catches my eye, reminding me of last week's lifeless, leathery spaghetti. I sigh as I get up to retrieve and untangle the mess, my mind enjoying a playful wander. Realizing I need a better storage system, I carelessly drop the confused cables and pick up my smartphone, heading over to the Amazon app. I begin scrolling—*Who knew there were gazillion ways to tame cable carnage? Wait. What's that in my checkout cart? Ooh—I should probably purchase that "Wine O'Clock" wall clock right now since the 29 percent discount could disappear in a New York minute.*

Reaching for my now lukewarm coffee, I make a mental note to get back to these ridiculously niggly tasks another time. My eyes scan back to my laptop, trying to recapture the thought of the report. I glance at my watch, and my heart sinks. An hour has passed, and I've achieved absolutely NADA. And my coffee tastes like cold, wet newspaper.

What on earth happened? Or, to be precise, what didn't?

How could I become so distracted as I settled down to draft my report? My mind was clearly multitasking but be damned if I could sync it with another body part to make something—*anything*—productive happen. Ian Haynes, a very wise man, once said, "When we jump from task to task, we aren't getting more done. In actuality, we're forcing our brains to constantly switch gears, working harder to do things at a lower level of quality and exhausting our mental reserves."

It can also be called the FAFF.

"Faff" is an informal British word that means to dither, flap, or fuss. If you say someone is faffing around, as the *Macmillan Dictionary* states, it can be that they invite unnecessary trouble involving something unimportant. Ouch. I affectionately label this phenomenon "the Frustrating Art of Fussing and Flapping."

I've spent much of my adult life perfecting the FAFF, and the older I get, the more I love it. I enjoy aimlessly scrolling through the house just as much as my smartphone, and I get immense pleasure from gliding (or sometimes hurtling) from one physical surface to another. I'll notice something that needs attention and think about it for a hot second before quickly moving on to the next distraction. I revel in the daydream until I get bored or sidetracked, and then my poor, sweet brain just hurts!

A Handbook for Sparking a Sassy Morning

It is the most frustrating conundrum, this faffing thing. But it got me thinking. If observing myself wandering somewhat pointlessly around the house brought me small moments of pleasure, could I turn it into a productive and loving ritual that could bring accomplishment and, therefore, an element of joy into my day? Could this help elevate my mojo?

I got to work. I honed in. I rethought the FAFF—and it was deliciously simple and satisfying.

The breakthrough for me was the series of small actions I took *before* beginning a task. It was much more than just checking off the to-do list. First, I took a notepad and wrote down all of the small, tedious, or forgettable tasks I could fill my brain with that were standing, lying, or dead before me as evidence of neglect. Then I chose one of these (small, tedious, forgettable) jobs that I knew I could complete within a few minutes. I threw on some music. I set the timer on my phone. Then I got down to business.

I vowed I would stay focused *on the task at hand* so I could finish it and maybe even beat the clock (I'm competitive like that). As I succeeded, I repeated the sequence with another chore on my list, setting a specific, brief period to complete it. I repeated this process again and again. Each of these undertakings was relatively easy and offered a strong sense of contentment once done.

For me, the success or the power of the FAFF lies within its *given timeframe*. By committing to a tiny task that you can complete in a few minutes—think thirty seconds to five minutes—you are compelled to streamline your thoughts and actions to get the job done. Otherwise, distraction and daydreaming can tiptoe in (and they deserve their own chapter, don't you think?).

I understood the importance of this when I absentmindedly forgot to push 'start' on my phone timer as I embarked upon tearing out keepable articles from a pile of old yet beloved fitness magazines. I began in earnest, flicking through, ripping pages, and discarding the rest until my mind wandered around the ten-minute mark and that feeling of "beige" crept in. I started losing interest, picking at my nails, wondering what on earth had happened to the timer.

Sweet reader, remember to set your alarm. Here's a double-whammy trick to address the 'in-case-I-forget' issue and inject some fun into your task: line up two of your all-time favorite songs and push play. Your task should be complete by the time the music fades out. It's simple, and it works.

Reframing small annoying tasks as self-care can help you see and value their importance. As I added this faffing ritual into my mornings, I discovered that restructuring small jobs this way brought great delight to my day. I was on to something. And completing this ritual within the first hour of my day when I had the most energy not only allowed me to feel fabulously fulfilled within a short time, but I actually had a practical household task crossed off my list before breakfast—now that's a first.

The FAFF shall now be known as "the Fabulous Art of Feeling Fulfilled!"

The reimagined FAFF can help you gain clarity through planned moments of what is needed and ultimately brings you into the present moment in a sublimely subtle way. It's a positive, purposeful, and productive practice where you make room for the smaller, seemingly less important, but hugely satisfying tasks. Yet, you don't distract yourself from more significant tasks requiring your laser focus. That's good news, as studies show that humans typically spend 25–50 percent of their time thinking about thoughts irrelevant to their current situation, which can lead to increased distractibility when performing tasks. Yikes!

Faff tasks should involve everyday chores or personal tasks rather than work-related or digital tasks like bill payments or virtual retail therapy. Call me old school but there's a satisfying touch of nostalgia in tackling hands-on tasks right where you are.

Humans can experience multiple feelings at once, but did you know that because fairies are so small, they only have room for one emotion at a time? It says so in *Peter Pan*. Imagine yourself as Tinkerbell, honing in on one tiny thought or feeling while sprinkling your fairy dust as you happily go about your faffing! Your task and timeframe are so small that it becomes your sole focus. You aim to finish the job before the dust settles. This small sense of achievement can lead to joy—and sometimes to reminiscing about a favorite childhood fairytale.

Inch Inside. Do you ever have outbreaks of procrastinitis? Think of a small, niggly task you've been putting off or have started but not yet completed.

Write the task here:

....

....

Ask yourself why you're resisting or procrastinating. What is holding you back?

Circle all that apply:
- Lack of motivation
- Poor time management
- Lack of time
- Low energy levels
- Environmental distractions
- Feeling of overwhelm
- Anxiety
- Other (write it here) ....

Using the task identified above, what next small concrete step could help move you closer to action? For example: *I will turn my phone to silent,* or *I'll reward myself with an extra ten minutes of "me" time.*

✎ *Write it here:*

....
....

Follow the Flow. Now, let's identify some projects for your future faff sessions.

✎ *Brainstorm a small, specific task that you'd like to fulfill next to whatever action words nudge you. Ensure that each task can be completed within five minutes or less.*

- ☐ Set up . . .
- ☐ Delete . . .
- ☐ Tidy . . .
- ☐ Change . . .
- ☐ Move . . .
- ☐ Refold . . .
- ☐ Declutter . . .
- ☐ Consolidate . . .
- ☐ Clean . . .
- ☐ Streamline . . .
- ☐ Sanitize . . .
- ☐ Untangle . . .
- ☐ Rearrange . . .
- ☐ Reorganize . . .

The Joyful Toolbox

The sweet spot is where inspiration thrives, and action takes flight. If you've ever been distracted by procrastination, know you're not alone. By following a few simple steps, you can find yourself so fulfilled that you'll want to dive into tasks with gusto again and again. With practice, you'll learn to anticipate and relish these moments, and each time will become easier because you genuinely enjoy it.

Let's explore practical ways to prepare for some faffing good times. First, ensure there are no interruptions in sight. Mute your phone, check that there are no upcoming meetings, confirm any small humans in the building are occupied, and there are no cheetahs under the bed . . . you get my drift.

When deciding on a task, start with a quick list of those bite-sized household chores, each taking five minutes or less. Select one from your lineup, or let your curiosity guide you and see what in your room or space calls out for your attention. Keeping your options open keeps the ritual fresh and smoothly transitions you from awareness to action.

The FAFF Plan:
- Choose your task.
- Set a clear timeframe.
- Round up your materials.
- Fire up that timer.
- Dive into action.

Examples of the reimagined FAFF
Sort, reorganize, tidy, rearrange, clean, change, declutter—and any other motivating verbs
- Rearrange a pile of books in a new and interesting way.
- Tidy shoes back onto a shelf.

- Change out your table centerpiece to reflect a new season.
- Move a piece of furniture to a new spot.
- Refold clothes in an untidy drawer.
- Declutter your coffee table.
- Sanitize your gadgets.
- Untangle your cords (damn it, just do this one, trust me).
- Write your to-do list on individual colored sticky notes and post them in a prominent place.
- Clean out your makeup drawer.
- Polish those lackluster kitchen appliances.
- Color-code your filing system for easier access.
- Tackle the junk drawer (sort *only* similar types of things if you know this requires more time).
- Streamline your spices.
- Consolidate first-aid supplies.
- Set up a jewelry storage system.
- Pick up and put away an annoying pile of clothes.

Arrive, anchor, and unearth your energy.

Summarize your intention for launching your FAFF practice.

....
....

List the materials and resources you will need.

....
....

✍ *What tweaks does your ritual need?*

....

....

✍ *What are you learning about yourself through this practice?*

....

....

Faffing: the delightful art of self-care that not only gets things done but also leaves us with that warm, fuzzy feeling inside! When we embrace the FAFF, we're actually tapping into our mojo and infusing meaning and productivity into a tiny slice of the day. This simple practice can bring us wee nuggets of joy instead of sucking the life out of us as we mindlessly browse our Amazon app.

JUICY SELF-JOURNALING
Release Your Real Self and Lose Your Mind

Dear Journal,
Thank you
for letting me inflict
upon you the grazes and
scuffs of my words. For holding
my dreams in your pages and gathering
my rage as I spill hot, salty tears. For embracing
wild, windblown memories that cast lasting
wrinkles on my heart. There are
answers in your silence—
sometimes too
loud to
hear.

I received my first diary as a gift on my thirteenth birthday. It had a hard maroon cover with *Diary* boldly engraved on the front in shiny gold. A recording log had become all the craze with my peers since we'd studied *The Diary of Anne Frank* in English class, and the quote, "because paper has more patience than people," became our resolute mantra. I couldn't wait to fill the gleaming white pages with all the gushings of a newly christened teenage girl.

I madly wrote about my crush on the pimply, brown-eyed boy with lashes longer than mine whom I sat across from in History class. I also found myself sharing stories about my quirky family (because, let's face it, all families are weird when you're thirteen). And then, there was the time I couldn't help but admire crazy kid Wayne Seaton when he gallantly offered to toast my ham and cheese sandwich on the open heater during art class.

As each adolescent year flew by, I was gifted a new diary, and I couldn't wait to pour my heart and soul into it. Under the warm glow of torchlight, I diligently scribbled away almost every night, documenting every twist and turn of my life—from the mundane to the momentous, even my own zombie apocalypses!

Now, looking back, I can't help but chuckle at my younger self. If I could turn back time, I'd probably give her a gentle nudge and say, "Hey, burning toast isn't really an art form, you know. And zombies? Well, they're just bad moments dressed in drag."

But those diaries were more than just a way to chronicle my teenage escapades. They were my safe haven, my free therapy, and my trusted confidants. As time passed, I became the CEO of countless therapy sessions with myself. What started as shy recounts and occasional teenage outbursts blossomed into a love affair with raw, descriptive narratives in my adult years. I began throwing my feelings around like confetti at a wedding in Tornado Valley, ferociously exploring my interior landscape with all the verve and adjectives I could muster. Over the decades, my newly coined "journal" became a wildly honest reflection of myself, capturing the essence of who I was and who I've become.

It got very juicy, indeed.

I have a confession. I love to hit things. I'm talking about boxing, the fast, furious, and fun activity that clears your mind and sculpts beautiful arms. I love how laser-focused attention is required as your mind-body connection creates momentum to get the most power out of each strike. Try punching for several minutes, and stress and energy melt away, leaving you with feelings of calm and well-being thanks to the happy hormone dopamine.

In this sense, journaling is like boxing and therapy, all wrapped up into one powerful duo. You show up in the moment as (emotional) energy is shifted to another object (a blank piece of paper, in this case), allowing you to unleash your inner power through writing. I love losing myself in the strikes and punches of words.

Journaling opens unimagined doors in our hearts and teaches us how it was, how it is now, and how it could be. For me, it is a gorgeous act of self-love and self-care because I have free rein to nurture my thoughts and become truly myself on those pages. My morning journaling ritual means I begin my day positively and with a grateful heart. It helps align my intentions and improve my focus while giving me pause to think about the day ahead.

When it comes to journaling, there are no strict rules. Your journal is yours to shape and mold, making it an empowering tool for manifesting abundance and joy in your life. It's been my faithful companion, helping me show up for myself time and time again, especially on days when life feels like a wild whirlwind. Julia Cameron's Morning Pages ritual, as shared in *The Artist's Way*, has been a game-changer for my journaling practice. Her simple yet powerful advice to put pen to paper daily has been a guiding light, helping me through fears, negativity, and mood swings, leading me to a place of positivity and action. Let it be your anchor, your sounding board, and your source of empowerment. As Julia Cameron says, "Daily morning writing can help us get to the other side," and she's absolutely right.

My journal is my entry point to release stress and anxiety, monitor progress, and continue to focus and stay motivated. Each of these elements offers a strong sense of mojo as I figure out my thoughts by collecting them in one place and feel empowered as I become curious about them. Ferris Bueller, in the classic movie of the same name, said, "Life moves pretty fast. If you don't stop and look around once in a while, you could miss it." Journaling gives me a moment to pause, reflect, examine the landscape, and recalibrate in a world that shows no signs of slowing down.

A Handbook for Sparking a Sassy Morning

Inch Inside. "Emotions can get in the way—or get *you* on the way." Mavis Mazhura, human behavior specialist.

🖊 *What makes you feel everything? Write down the first thought that pops into your head next to each of these words.*

Curious ....
Vulnerable ....
Badass ....
Exhausted ....
Shameless ....
Paralyzed ....
Blissful ....

Follow the Flow. Choose one of your responses above and connect it to a specific moment in your life.

🖊 *Write a short entry about what, why, and how you felt. Be 'bronest' (brutally honest). Go on, feel all the feels!*

....
....
....
....
....

The Joyful Toolbox

Have you ever experienced a fleeting moment of brilliance, only for the idea to vanish before you could grasp it? Or perhaps you jotted down a stroke of genius on a scrap of paper, only to misplace it moments later? In this toolbox, I'll share three playful methods I use to capture and preserve my thoughts.

Smile if you're someone who talks aloud to themselves. I'm a shameless "talker-to-myself" and it happens everywhere and all the time. There's something liberating about hashing out arguments, exploring ideas, and venting whatever's on my mind—it's just between my big mouth and sweet little brain. It's like having my own private sanctuary of thoughts and musings! When I delved into journaling, I knew it had to be something super special to keep me coming back every day. That's when a great idea came to mind, inspired by my habit of talking to myself—I call it the *Talk Report Technique,* a journaling approach that's been a game-changer for me and still serves me well today.

I was on a neighborhood power walk, with my 'Fierce Women' playlist blaring in my ears when a tiny, yet thrilling, idea struck me about my recent art project. The tune of "Unstoppable" by Sia, playing in the background seemed to fuel the spark, making it grow into something bigger. I knew I had to take action before it slipped away. Remembering the voice memo app on my phone I paused the music and excitedly recorded my ideas on the spot. The mix of fresh air, empowering music, and feel-good hormones made my thoughts flow effortlessly. I was unstoppable! When I returned home, I listened to the recording and jotted down notes in my journal. I was super-chuffed that I could use my phone for being a creative genius on the go. Who knew my trusty device could be my creative companion?

This type of one-on-one conference is great for when you're out and about or on the fly and don't have time to collect paper to write. Pop on your headphones, and you could be on a call with a friend; it's super discreet. I also use this method to have that challenging discussion with myself. I even use it for "cralking"—simultaneously crying, talking, and walking. This type of vulnerability feels liberating to me. On a side note, if you choose to revisit your recordings later to mull over or take physical notes, that's fantastic! If you prefer to delete them afterward, that's quite all right too.

Freedom Writer is another of my favorite ways of journaling, where you start writing whatever comes into your mind. It's an open book; only your imagination can hold you back. Whether your first entries are one word or one hundred, whether you find an old, unused notebook or invest in a fancy journal that offers a structure, a blank page is all you need to get started. I like decorating a notebook's cover with a favorite inspirational quote or affirmation, so I'm motivated from the get-go. Keep your journal in a place where you can access it easily. I find that setting out one of my favorite gel pens on my desk is helpful as a reminder to grab my journal. If you need extra motivation to start, try setting a goal to write continuously for a specified number of pages or set a time frame and let your thoughts flow, unedited, onto the page.

Ever found yourself staring at a blank page, struggling to gather your thoughts? Sometimes, all you need is a little nudge to kick-start your creativity. That's where *Romp with a Prompt* comes in—a simple sentence that can ignite the storyteller within you.

Use these ten prompts to get started. Stick with one for a week and watch how your thoughts and feelings evolve, or choose a new one each day. Just jot down the starter in your journal and let it guide your thoughts.

1. My favorite way to spend the day . . .
2. If I could change anything about my life . . .
3. How I might overcome a challenge I'm facing right now . . .

4. A mistake people often make about me . . .
5. What keeps me up at night worrying . . .
6. The kindest thing I can do for myself when I'm in physical or emotional pain . . .
7. A past challenge that turned out to be a blessing in disguise . . .
8. Something I disagree with, and how this triggers me . . .
9. The magic power I would like to have and how I would use it . . .
10. Ten things that always make me feel better, no matter what . . .

Returning to your journal is like unlocking a memory treasure chest filled with those 'aha' moments that might have slipped your mind. Reading your entries in the moment lets you reflect on the spot, and returning to them later reveals new perspectives and hidden insights. Or, you can leave your words undisturbed, treating your journal like a time capsule. When you're ready to dive in, it's like playing 'face-emoji,' with smirks, furrowed brows, and moments of introspection as you randomly flip open a page.

Arrive, anchor, and unearth your energy.

Summarize your intention for launching your journaling practice.

....
....

List the materials and resources you will need.

....
....

> ✒ *What tweaks does your ritual need?*
> ....
> ....
>
> ✒ *What are you learning about yourself through this practice?*
> ....
> ....

If it sounds daring and wanton to release your authentic self and lose your mind—well, it is! Journaling grants us moments to dream, to weave ideas into plans and goals, all of which can find expression within the pages of your own voluptuous volume. It's the perfect way to get in touch with your mojo, and there are countless ways to do it. Your one goal with journaling, sweet reader, is simply to start because, as the authors of our own stories, our tales are too juicy not to tell!

GROOM YOUR GOAL-TENTION

Ignite Your Intention to Action

> **Be**
> *still,*
> *become*
> *perfectly present.*
> *Weigh your why and grow*
> *your intention. Dream breathtakingly big.*
> *Determine your destination. Birth*
> *your purpose and set your*
> *goal-tention.*

It is a cold gray winter's day in the exercise yard. My feet slip slightly on the wet grass, and my breath makes fragile steam rings as I perform the last push-up and move into a plank position. My workout spot is in the farthest concrete corner of the complex, well away from all other humans in their masks walking the perimeter of the enclosure. Jet lag still has its blanket wrapped tightly around me as I begin day three of two weeks of captivity in a quarantined hotel in New Zealand.

    As I near the end of my plank time, I see them: a pair of large army boots, sandy beige and highly polished. They park themselves inches away from my splayed hands and rigid body. "Excuse me, ma'am," the young voice north of the boots whispers. "You can't do that."

    My eyes become squinty, and I suck in my cheeks, my poker face about to become very expressive. This is the *third* time I have been chewed out for either jogging, squatting, or throwing a few burpees around in *the exercise yard*. Did my brain abort the plane mid-flight and parachute itself to la-la land? I clearly missed the memo regarding the "E-word," which, I have since found out, has been reduced to a brisk quarantine walk at best. Frustration lands on my aching shoulders. My hands and feet cement themselves to the concrete below while my mind and mouth are one sound bite away from a snarky outburst.

Balancing in the plank position, I'm deep in thought, strategizing to prevent exercise yard meltdowns and other potential challenges. It's no walk in the park, believe me. As I center my mind, I summon my well-crafted quar-intent (a little wordplay I came up with for setting intentions during quarantine). After brushing off the mental debris and ego dust, I push myself up and confront the situation head-on.

"BOY, you must be tired of being the exercise yard enforcer," I quip, flashing a mischievous grin at the young army recruit. "Seems like you've drawn the short straw, trying to keep us from our workouts!" But right then, I resolved to brighten his day with a splash of sunshine and a dash of kindness.

Why do we often have the best intentions, but following them through can feel like assembling Ikea furniture without a manual? Are they just heat-of-the-moment promises to ourselves? Why is it so hard to make them stick?

Consider this: We humans love to binge on intentions in the New Year, only to fall by the wayside by mid-January. We give up, move on, and even forget what we planned in the first place. As I've learned, this is a surefire way to lose your mojo.

Rewind to my scenario in the exercise yard. Would my quarantine intention of cultivating kindness hit the mark? Could I reach my goal and truly practice some loving-kindness? Or was it just wishful thinking? Jennifer Williamson, the writer of *Healing Brave Manifesto*, has a beautiful saying: "Intention is more than wishful thinking—it's willful direction." I love this analogy. So, what exactly is intention, and how can we make willful direction happen?

An intention is essentially a commitment to a state we'd like to be in—of how we want to live or feel as we show up and move throughout our day. It's about the energy we want to attract and the kind of person we want to be *right now*. Intention is the process we go through until we get to what we concretely achieve through a specific action. This action then becomes a *goal* set in the future and describes an endpoint for a desired result. When we're intentional about something, we focus on the present moment. My frustration during my stint in the exercise yard boosted my resolve to act right then. To cultivate kindness was a genuine purpose-based desire I wanted to nurture in my day-to-day life during quarantine. "To greet the guards with a friendly, uncondescending smile" was an action to move me closer to fulfilling this intention.

Omar Itani, the writer of *The Optimist,* aptly summed up the difference between intention and goals.

"If goals are rooted in your tomorrow, intentions are rooted in your today.

If goals are where you want to take your life, intentions are who you're actively becoming.

If goals are fixated on what's next, intentions keep you focused on what's now.

If goals are about a destination, intentions are about a direction."

So, what then is a "goal-tention"?
Sweet reader, it's a concept I've crafted, merging the "now" with the "what will be" into a practical idea. Think of it as aligning your inner compass with a goal that truly vibes with you. When our intentions and goals are crystal clear, our mojo gets a power boost, moving us toward greater clarity, self-assurance, and joy.

Consider each morning as a chance to check in with yourself and set an intention for the day. Some days, you might wake up with a clear purpose in mind, while on others, you'll need a few moments to sit with your thoughts. Your intention might remain consistent for several days or weeks, or it could change more frequently. But taking small, achievable steps toward fulfilling your goal will turn your aspirations into realities. This simple approach brings a breath of fresh air, empowering you to make meaningful progress toward your daily aspirations.

One of the first things I do to kick-start my morning mojo is to focus on my day's intention. This sets up my day with a trajectory that aligns with what's important to me. It's simple and easy to do. Let's try it together.

Inch inside. Take a deep breath and visualize how you want today to unfold.

What are you longing for? What do you want to be more of? Check one of the statements below. You can also write your own.

- ☐ Seek calm
- ☐ Enjoy the journey
- ☐ Create momentum
- ☐ Trust myself
- ☐ Rest
- ☐ Make things happen

- ☐ Invite peace
- ☐ Cultivate kindness
- ☐ Surprise myself
- ☐ Keep it simple
- ☐ Have the courage
- ☐ ....

Identifying your "why" behind an intention paves the way for future action because achieving that goal becomes much easier once you focus on who you want to *be*.

Write today's intention and say why this state of mind, attitude, or feeling is important to you.

....
....
....
....

> **Follow the Flow.** Energy is infused into intention by creating a small, concrete goal, so it becomes an action and a positive step toward self-love.
>
> 🖋 *Write one small, specific, achievable action step toward your intention.*
>
> ....

Some examples of my past goal-tentions:
- Value my time without technology by detaching myself for one hour from all devices.
- Make time to relax and unwind by scheduling 30 minutes to reconnect with my sister.
- Follow my bliss and have a dance party for one just because it makes me happy.
- Get out of my comfort zone and post that new YouTube video I've been holding back on.
- Let go of that nagging feeling by scheduling the overdue dentist appointment.
- Face that potentially prickly phone call by reframing my thinking into a vibe of, "I've got this!"
- Get some exercise by planning an impromptu run through a new neighborhood.
- Stop, close my eyes, and rest for ten minutes.

The Joyful Toolbox

You've identified your goal-tention, but the ritual doesn't finish there. It's the follow-through and manifestation that bring about change. This is where you need to be firm with yourself about not forgetting what you have set.

How can you do that? Three simple steps include *writing it down, placing it in a visible space* where you can be reminded of it throughout your day, and then *reflecting on your progress* before you tuck yourself into bed at night. This will often direct you to the next small step of repeating any goal-tention that is unmet or setting a new one. Take time to think about not only your desired outcome but the process of *how you are becoming*, as this will keep your intention and goal aligned.

Who doesn't love both the functional and the fabulous? I'm a visual person who finds inspiration in colors and beauty while keeping things practical. Here are two ways to track goal-tention that check these boxes. Maybe they will resonate with you, or perhaps you will create your own method to suit your time, energy, personality, and motivation.

Take a colorful Post-it note, jot down your goal-tention, and stick it in a place where you can see it and be reminded throughout the day. I write my intention on several Post-its and stick them all over the house—on the oil diffuser at my desk, the bathroom mirror, and the washing machine (very strategic, I know). At the end of the day, I'll gather them up and pop them onto my passion board, which is simply a corkboard containing collected pictures, poems, and notes of my hopes and daydreams.

Decorate the cover of a plain notebook with an affirmation that vibrates with you and log your daily goal-tentions inside. Mine is a cute, teeny, student notepad, perfect for the one-goal-tention-per-page effect.

It's kept on my office desk and is the first thing I see, and therefore reach for when I sit down at my desk each morning. Oh, and if you want to keep a stash of shiny gold-star stickers tucked into the back of your notepad—you know, the same kind that kindergarten teachers use to motivate five-year-olds—that's a lovely way to reward yourself on your goal-tention journey.

Arrive, anchor, and unearth your energy.

🖋 *Summarize your intention for launching your goal-tention practice.*

....
....

🖋 *List the materials and resources you will need.*

....
....

🖋 *What tweaks does your ritual need?*

....
....

🖋 *What are you learning about yourself through this practice?*

....
....

"Weigh your why and grow your intention." It's like a little pause to reflect on your true motivations. Living by your values creates a path where mojo naturally adds joy and purpose to your days. There's really no better moment than the present to make your real intentions happen—because, unlike the past or the future, now is the only time there is.

Body

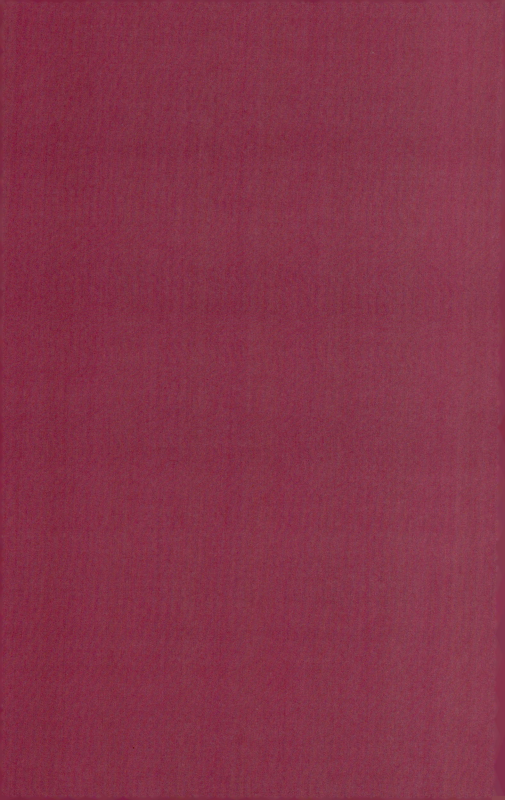

MANIFEST A MOVE
Body Language for Moving Vividly

Sway

and shimmy.
Push, pull, reach, and rise.
Undulate, stretch, cavort, and flex.
Lift, vibrate, extend, and sink into
your signature movement.
Bless your bewitching
body. Be in motion
for it aches to
feel truly
alive.

It was a harmless flirt. I just *had* to own the hot-pink Lycra leotard seductively laid out before me. I sighed with delight as my hands tenderly touched the teeny, tiny costume. It came with the whole shebang—matching slouchy leg warmers, neon leggings, a wide, black stretchy belt, and those oh-so-chic terry cloth wristbands. I was nineteen, and this was my first act of expressing my freedom. Having recently joined the YMCA, I was aching to play the part, to dress to express my newfound commitment to exercise, and to the world of making it on my own. I signed the check, tucked the package under my arm, and left the shop positively glowing with badassery.

Blame it on the iconic Jane-Fonda-inspired trend of the times, but I proudly paraded my thirty-centimeter, ridiculously expensive strip of spandex for "the Movement." I felt fit and cute in my sassy suit. It powered me through many aerobics classes and let me relax in style on the very fashionable motorized tables of the times that would gently move and stretch my body while I thought of Mother England.

But my ankles itched. I'm sure I had crotch cleavage, and my cinched waist was hotter than a shirtless Michael Landon in a *Little House on the Prairie* episode. I was chafed and probably one aerobic step away from a nasty yeast infection. But that was back then. Mercifully, those moving machines went out of business within a hot minute, and spandex got better. Now it can be stretched up to almost five times its original length.

I love that feeling when I consciously propel my body into action. It feels good to know the muscles are hard at work, my body is getting stronger and more limber, and I'm paving the way for more mobile elder years. Lifting weights and dancing are two of my favorite ways to move.

What's your ultimate go-to for staying active and having fun? Are you a cardio queen, a gym junkie, or a Zen goddess? How about shaking it up with a dance session? Or are you all about those invigorating neighborhood power walks, or playing frisbee or soccer in the backyard with your mini-crew? And who could resist the charm of those vintage toning tables? They teleport us back to the good old days of quick workouts (or maybe we were just secretly relaxing without anyone knowing!).

Let me ask you, how does your body feel when your feet hit the ground first thing in the morning? Energized, limber, and ready to start the day? Are your mind and body in sync, or do they need to discuss the situation over coffee first? After seven or eight hours cocooned in dreamland, is your gorgeous body aching to unfold and gently spread her wings before taking flight?

It's normal for our body to feel a little tight after waking. As we move along the spectrum of life, we lose bone density, especially leading up to, during, and after the mind-boggling period of menopause. The bones lose calcium and other minerals, joints become stiffer and less flexible, and muscles can lose their tone.

But it's not all gloomisery!

Movement is the medicine that can set us on the path to vitality. Maintaining strength, balance, and flexibility through exercise is one of the best ways to slow or prevent problems with the musculoskeletal system. Whatever our age, there's no reason why we can't enter each new year and phase of our life feeling fit, healthy, and vibrant. And think about this: When we get moving in the morning, it prepares us both physically and mentally by getting the blood flowing and creating positive energy to launch us into our day—so our mojo gets a workout too!

Perhaps you're feeling optimistic about a current fitness regime.

Or maybe you have yet to find an activity that really moves you.

Stay with me, sweet reader. When we feel good about ourselves, it shows in our physical body, smiles, eyes, and how we carry ourselves. When our confidence or motivation fades, it can be said we've momentarily lost our mojo—our desire to get up, show up, and find those moments of joy. For me, one of the most exciting elements of mojo is confidence. Who doesn't feel a little more badass and energized after a workout, a walk, or hitting the dance floor?

For those of you who haven't historically had positive experiences with keeping your body strong and limber, I see you, too. I've had to work around two hip replacements and numerous other surgeries, which sometimes had me down-and-out. But our bodies are resilient, and if we listen to them closely, we can work around our limitations and celebrate what they can do. By bringing some sass and a playful approach toward movement, I hope you'll feel encouraged to give your body the extra attention it surely deserves.

Roadblocks

If exercise is so important, then what holds us back? We say that we're too tired—even though we just woke up; we declare we're too out of shape—so we need to wait until that shape changes; we gripe about how life is busy enough already—there's absolutely no room for another thing, my dear!

Maybe you used to exercise when you were younger—when you had more time—but now, raising a family, attending to a dog and two cats, and caring for an aging parent can change your priorities. Exercise is an indulgence, after all!

As one of my clients, Louise was the ultimate 'giver of energy.' She poured herself into charities, family, friends, church, and community, but her own energy reserves were running precariously low. Exhausted and disheartened, she sought fitness coaching with me, determined to reclaim her vitality. Together, we embarked on a journey of small, intentional steps. Louise began by scheduling short bursts of exercise into her daily routine—five minutes of morning stretches and fifteen minutes of walking three times a week. These small steps became a turning point for her. Her zest for life started to bounce back, and she gradually added strength training and established regular fitness routines.

With each milestone, Louise's transformation was evident. Not only did she shed those extra pounds, but her vibrant and fun-loving spirit returned, accompanied by a newfound sense of confidence. The change in her was palpable. Louise had unlocked her mojo by making herself a priority. Together, we proved that self-care isn't selfish—it's the key to offering your best self to the world. A few minutes a day can truly make all the difference, and Louise's story serves as a powerful reminder of the transformative power of self-care.

So, sweet reader, this is your cue.

Once you begin, momentum will follow, and before you know it, paying attention to how your body moves will become a consistent and joyful part of your day. Start right where you are—yes—even if you're still in your cozy little crib wanting an extra ten minutes of dreamtime. You just need a plan.

I have clients who swear by a morning yoga routine to prep for those not-so-Zen moments. Then there are the early birds who kick-start their day with a walk or jog. As for me, my early morning groove begins with easing my perpetually creaky hips with gentle stretches or perhaps a solo dance party to get my blood pumping and mojo in high gear. The winning formula? Choose something that genuinely lights you up—and make it a daily dose of joy.

Inch Inside. Think of how your body felt when you got up today.
Where do you fall on the spectrum?
Meh .... Fab!

Think about your current attitudes and beliefs around exercise. Go on, be ridiculously honest.

Finish these sentences.
- Moving my body feels

....

- Exercise to me means

....

- Something that holds me back from exercise is

....

- What motivates me the most to exercise is
  ....
- My favorite way to move my body is
  ....

Follow the Flow. We all have different reasons for exercising or wanting to start an exercise program.

✎ *Check the movement goals that are important to you.*
☐ Increase energy levels
☐ Feel better and improve overall health
☐ Increase strength, flexibility, or cardiovascular fitness
☐ The fun factor
☐ Improve mood and ability to cope with stress
☐ Longevity
☐ Other ....

✎ *Take the goal that resonates the most with you and write how you could inch towards this by incorporating movement into your day.*
....
....
....

The Joyful Toolbox

This toolbox adapts to your fitness journey, making it easy to match your morning vibes with the movement you need.

The Wake-Up Series consists of four simple exercise routines designed to energize you in minutes. You don't need much to begin with—your bed, a chair, or a cozy nook will do the trick.

Don't sweat it if you're new to some of these exercises. Begin with one or two stretches or body-weight moves. As you get the hang of it, gradually add more. If you're just starting out, ease into it gently and feel free to do fewer reps or hold poses briefly. And for those looking for an extra challenge, go ahead and push yourself with more reps or run through the routine again. It's up to you, and the possibilities are wide open. And as you dive into these energizing routines, keep in mind that every step you take brings you closer to a healthier, more energized version of yourself.

Workout Routines

Wake Up and Unfold consists of six stretches to limber up the major muscles of your body. All you need is a flat surface and a small space. Hold each pose for ten to twenty seconds. Follow the exercises for a gentle flow, or choose individual poses that resonate with you.

WAKE UP AND UNFOLD

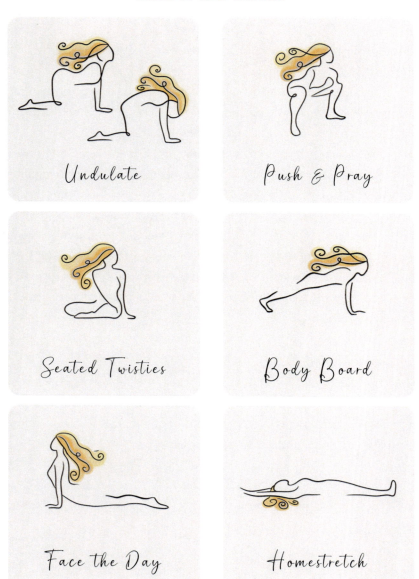

Undulate: On all fours, inhale as you drop the belly and lift your head. Exhale and round the spine and lower your head.

Push & Pray: Stand with a wide stance, feet slightly turned outwards. Lower your butt toward the ground and gently use the elbows to push your knees out.

Seated Twisties: Sitting on the bed with your legs crossed, place your right hand on your left knee and gently twist your body to the left. Repeat on the other side.

Body Board: Start on all fours on the floor with hands stacked directly under the shoulders and your knees stacked directly under the hips. Push up into a high plank position, squeeze heels and glutes together, and draw your navel to your spine.

Face the Day: Lie on your stomach and place your hands flat beneath your shoulders. Tuck your elbows into your sides and gently raise your head and chest, lifting your torso.

Homestretch: Lie on your back, reach the arms overhead, clasp your fingers together, and wriggle your body, so you feel it elongate and stretch.

Wake Up Between the Sheets is a cheeky option for bedheads who prefer to get moving while still under the covers. Why not! Make sure you have enough space to perform these exercises. Inviting a bedmate is optional. ;)

Follow the progression of exercises, holding each pose for ten to twenty seconds.

Don't Mess With My Mojo

WAKE UP BETWEEN THE SHEETS

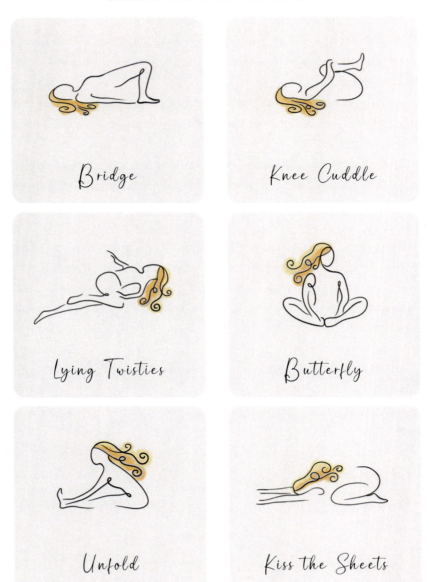

Bridge: Lie on your back and gently raise your hips to create a straight line from the knees to the shoulders. Squeeze your core and pull your belly button back toward the spine.

Knee Cuddle: Lie on your back and bring both knees toward the chest, wrapping your arms around both shins. Squeeze gently.

Lying Twisties: From the knee cuddle pose, release your arms and let both knees fall to one side, straightening your lower leg while planting your shoulders square onto the mattress. Turn your neck to gaze toward the opposite side. Swap sides.

Butterfly: In a seated position, bring the soles of your feet to touch, allowing the knees to fall open away from each other.

Unfold: Sit up with your back straight, legs straight out in front, and feet flexed. Raise your arms above your head while inhaling. Exhale as you bend at the hips and reach your arms toward your toes.

Kiss the Sheets: Kneel and sit on your ankles. Lean forward, keeping your butt on the heels while resting your forehead on the bed. Move your arms out in front of you, palms facing down. Inhale and exhale slowly and deeply.

Wake Up And be Lightweight is a body-weight circuit including strength and cardio exercises that will get your blood pumping. You will need access to a raised surface such as a chair, bed, or step. Perform ten to fifteen repetitions of each exercise (count both sides as one rep). Repeat the circuit two to three times.

WAKE UP AND BE LIGHTWEIGHT

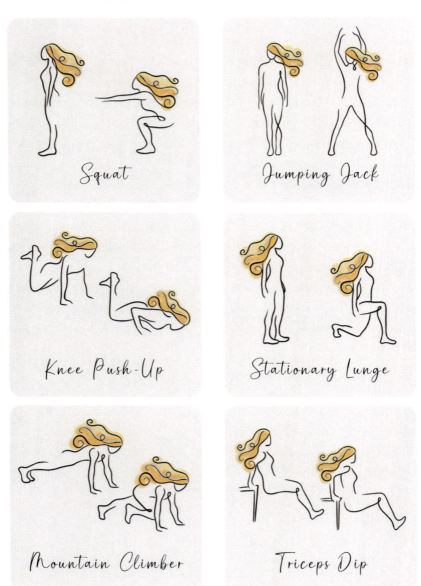

Squat: Stand with your feet shoulder-width apart and turned out slightly. Raise your arms out in front of you and lower your butt until your thighs are parallel to the floor. Pause, then return to the starting position.

Jumping Jack: Bend your knees slightly and jump into the air. As you jump, land with your feet about shoulder-width apart. Stretch your arms out and over your head. Jump back to your starting position.

Knee Push-Up: Kneel on the floor, extend your arms, and put your hands shoulder-width apart on the floor in front of you. Tighten your abdominals while you bend your arms, lowering your torso as much as possible. Push back up by straightening your arms (you can also do this exercise against the wall).

Stationary Lunge: Stand with your feet hip-distance apart, then take a large step forward with one foot. Lower the back knee to a ninety-degree angle so both knees are bent, then press up to start position and repeat—swap legs after desired repetitions.

Mountain Climber: Start from a high plank position with hands stacked directly under the shoulders. Drive one knee forward toward the chest while engaging the abdominals. Repeat the movement on the other leg, alternating legs and speeding up your movements.

Triceps Dip: Place your hands behind you onto a chair or step, so your fingers face forward. Extend your legs and bend your elbows, lowering your body towards the floor. Push yourself back to the starting position.

Wake Up and Groove is exactly that and doesn't need an explanation. Shimmy out of bed, sweet reader! Line up your favorite song or two on your smartphone, pop on some headphones, and sway, gyrate, or stamp your feet to the beat as you unleash your inner goddess.

There are several ways to approach these individual routines: *By working on a single routine for the entire week,* you'll become familiar with the movements and track your progress with ease. Make it a well-rounded fitness journey by *alternating days between a stretch sequence and an energizing routine,* achieving a nice balance of cardio, strength, and stretching. You have the freedom to *mix and match* exercises from each routine and end with a fabulous dance party! These routines can *complement your existing fitness program* or introduce a refreshing change, if you're ready to try something new.

Challenge yourself by stepping out of your comfort zone. If you're a gym enthusiast, explore "Wake Up and Unfold" for a fresh twist. Pilates lovers, don't miss out on a "Wake Up and Groove" party. Each routine can be a complete journey on its own, or simply choose the exercises that suit your body's needs on any given day. You do you!

Trust your body; it'll guide you.

Arrive, anchor, and unearth your energy.

Summarize your intention for launching your movement practice.

....
....

List the resources you will need.

....
....

What tweaks does your ritual need?

....
....

> ✒ *What are you learning about yourself through this practice?*
> ....
> ....

Manifest your move, energize your mojo, and seize the day, sweet reader. Exercise isn't just about taking care of your body; it's about infusing your life with joy and vitality. And when you sync your body with heart, mind, and spirit-loving rituals like journaling, meditation, and gratitude, you're setting the stage for a vibrant and fulfilling life. Celebrate your prime real estate—your gorgeous body—and let her be your daily dose of joy and motivation.

THE NAKED SMOOTHIE
Strip It Down and Suck It Up

Awaken
your senses.
Take yourself on
a tantalizing tropical trip,
taste the laid-back island vibe.
Climb aboard a flying carpet to the
intoxicating spice markets of magical Marrakesh.
Get Zen amongst the vibrant rice fields of Bali.
Wherever your tastebuds wander,
surrender to a moment
of wellness
in every
sip.

The first—ahem—smoothie I ever made was quite by accident, a very long time ago, before smoothies were even a thing. I was in cahoots with Kate, my crazy cousin-in-crime. Our cake-making debut was staged on the linoleum floor of the floral-wallpapered kitchenette of 10 Gardener Street.

The intention was to make a delicious chocolate cake for our grandad and present it to him for his birthday. We waited patiently until all responsible adults had left the building to mow the lawn and hang out the washing, as we say in New Zealand, and we got to work. Riffling through the kitchen cupboards and drawers, we pulled out bowls, spatulas, wooden spoons, and measuring cups. We collected baking supplies, and to our surprise, some not-so-baking foodstuffs joined the party too!

Our concoction had all the flavors and portions that two ten-year-olds could delight in. Copious amounts of sugar and cocoa came first. We then added a generous dollop or two of mayonnaise and all the leftover mashed potatoes from last night's dinner (for a creamy texture). In the murky recesses of the fridge, we discovered a half-drunk can of Fanta, and that became the highlight of our adventure. The mere thought of a fizzy cake made us squeal with delight! Of course, we couldn't forget the essentials—flour and eggs—because even ten-year-olds know you can't make a cake without those.

As we decanted and dissolved, stirred and spilled (a lot!), the kitchen soon resembled the aftermath of a toddler's tea party, to which Freddy Kruger had invited himself. Our cake batter resembled curdled sludge that even made the cat cringe. We tossed everything into the mighty Kitchen Wizz food processor. With sticky fingers and hopeful hearts, we blended and blitzed. Our proud little faces were so sure our cake creation would rise triumphantly. Let's push pause right there.

Unlike with my cake-making debut, no cooking is required with a smoothie. I compare it to drinking a gourmet fruit salad through a straw! The term "smoothie" was branded by the creator of the Smoothie King franchise in the 1970s, a guy called Steve Kuhnau. Back in the day, my mother was like a dating detective. She'd warn me about those sneaky smoothies—boys with not-so-great intentions. "Stay away!" she'd say—but I digress.

Having grown up with extreme food allergies and unable to enjoy the popular milkshakes his friends relished, Kuhnau, a nurse at the time, replicated his own version using fruit, protein sources, and ice. He began to thrive from consuming these drinks and encouraged his patients to try his concoctions. They began to see a positive effect on their health—and the rest, as they say, is history.

I've always been on the search to identify, create, and enjoy foods that make me feel good and that are also good for me. Smoothies—of the drinkable kind—check that box, as they can be a divinely delicious and nutritious part of your diet. I love that feeling of being fulfilled—literally and figuratively—by the power of this mighty and versatile drink. When we nourish our body with the goodness it deserves, that's mojo!

In my quest for nutrient-dense food, I discovered that smoothies are the perfect way to *increase our daily intake of fruits and veggies.* If you find it a mission to get enough fresh produce into your diet by blending fruits and vegetables, you are not only stepping up your daily quota into one smart drink but also allowing your body to absorb more nutrients. Research shows that by pulverizing produce, a plant's cell walls are broken down, resulting in easier digestion. And just in case you're gagging with an underwhelming sense to partake, a smoothie can disguise the taste of any vegetable because of all the other super-fun ingredients combined. Breathe a sigh of relief, sweet reader.

Who has time to whip up and create breathtaking breakfasts that deserve a spot on the next Netflix cooking show? Store-bought versions contain a lot of sugar and calories, so I prefer to create my own concoctions. Whisking up a spectacular and satisfying brekkie in a glass within minutes is often my favorite way to start the day. I love that it's a purposeful act of *self-love*. In this chapter, you'll learn about the power of smoothie packs—prepping ingredients in advance—saving you time and headaches when scrambling for something quick and easy to prepare.

So, *what* makes a smoothie truly awesome and healthy? Sweet reader, the world is your oyster! Let's start with the three macronutrients—the essential food groups our body needs most to keep us feeling at our optimal best. By incorporating carbohydrates in the form of fruits and veggies, lean protein, and healthy fats, you'll get a power-packed dose of nutrition that will energize you and keep you satisfied. And to add a delightful twist, why not throw in some herbs and spices for a sweet, smooth celebration of flavors?

Let's take a closer look. Carbohydrates are the powerhouse of our body, providing essential energy, and fruits and veggies are two of the healthiest carbs because they're packed with vitamins and minerals. Protein steps in as the muscle-builder and the guardian of our brain and nervous system, delivering those crucial amino acids, which are like the essential Lego pieces that our body uses to build and repair proteins. And don't forget about the superpower of healthy fats, essential for cell function, energy reserves, and safeguarding our precious organs. All these amazing macros team up in the fantastic smoothie.

The Library of Lusciousness
By following one easy plan, you have total control over what goes into your smoothies. With your blender ready, add one ingredient from each of the following categories. Start with a *liquid base* followed by a portion of fresh or frozen *fruit and veggies*. Add your *protein, fats, herbs, and spices*. A *sweet little chaser* is optional but rather luscious in small doses. Before serving, you may like to choose a *topper* to sprinkle over your smoothie because then it's a party!

Please note that this is not a complete list of ingredients, so feel free to add your favorites.

Build your Smoothie

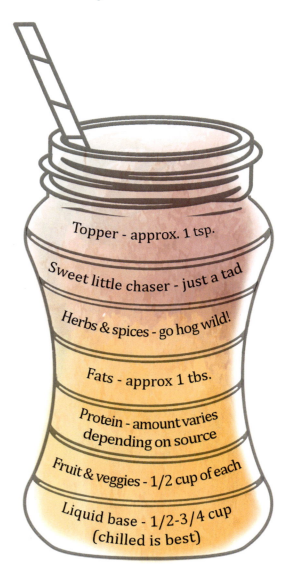

A Handbook for Sparking a Sassy Morning

Ingredients & Quantities

LIQUID BASE
H$_2$O or coconut water
nondairy milk
(almond, soy, coconut, etc.)
low-fat milk
100 % pure fruit
or veggie juice
unsweetened iced tea
or coffee

FRUIT
raspberries, blueberries
strawberries
mango, banana
cantaloupe, kiwi
apple, peach, apricot
pineapple
tangerine or orange

VEGGIES
raw zucchini, broccoli
cucumber, cauliflower
cooked pumpkin
sweet potato, beets
carrots, raw kale
spinach
collard greens

PROTEIN
protein powder
(whey or plant) - 1 serve
cottage cheese - 1/4c
silken or soft tofu - 1/4c
unsweetened yogurt
(Greek, or dairy-free) - 1/2 c
quinoa, cooked - 1/4c
tahini - 1 tbs.

FATS
nuts & nut butter
(almond, peanut
walnut, cashew, pecan)
seeds
(pumpkin
sunflower, chia, flax)
oils
(coconut, olive) -1 tsp.
avocado – ½c

HERBS & SPICES
cinnamon, turmeric
nutmeg, ginger
cayenne pepper
mint, basil
cilantro
vanilla extract
pumpkin pie spice

SWEET LITTLE CHASERS
1 Medjool date,
pitted & chopped
a drizzle of honey
or maple syrup
dried fruit,
chopped - 1 tbs.

TOPPER
granola, cacao nibs,
bee pollen,
flaked or shredded
unsweetened coconut
lemon or orange zest
crushed pistachios

Become your own smoothie master-chef
You don't need much to start, but an electric blender combines and mixes the ingredients into a smooth consistency. My compact Magic Bullet is perfect for making single servings. It's affordable and easy to set up, as well as clean. If you don't have access to a blender, although there's a bit more womanpower involved, you can hand-blend very ripe fruits and soft vegetables in a bowl using the back of a wooden spoon, a potato masher, or a fork. Add to a shaker cup, secure the lid, and start shaking—the shaker ball will help break down and mix the ingredients. It's a great workout—trust me.

To continue with the blender method, I first add most of the liquid base to the blender cup, followed by the fruits and vegetables. In goes protein, healthy fats, and unlimited herbs or spices, as these magical little boosters add to the flavor of any smoothie. They are excellent sources of nutrients needed for our well-being. You may want to use a smidgen of natural sweetener, but remember, a little goes a long way. Finally, I add the rest of the liquid to ensure a smooth consistency. Blend the ingredients for around sixty seconds, then pour your drink into your favorite vessel. I love my oversized plastic wine goblet I keep for this occasion. Lastly, sprinkle on your topping of choice, which looks visually appealing and can elevate a smoothie to something extraordinary. Reach for an environmentally friendly straw—I love bamboo—and sip away!

Inch Inside. Smoothies are a fun way of getting the nutrients our body needs, which is a loving act of self-care. What would you choose if there were no limits or restrictions to what you could put in your *ultimate smoothie*?

✒ *List the ingredients.*

....
....
....

Follow the Flow. Create your own smoothie using ingredients you love from the smoothie formula provided in this chapter, or add your own.

✒ *Select one ingredient from each category below and write it into the box. Don't forget to give your smoothie a name.*

Liquid base	Fruit	Veggies	Protein
Fats	Herbs & spices	Sweet little chaser	Topper

My signature smoothie is called

....

The Joyful Toolbox

Step into the vibrant world of smoothie creations, sweet reader, where your imagination is the only limit. Building your unique signature smoothie, as we did in the previous exercise, is a great place to discover what flavors tickle your taste buds.

Have fun with these travel-inspired recipes. (Try closing your eyes as you sip, it's a mini-vacation in your mind where you can manifest your next getaway.) Whether you're in the mood for an adventurous kick, a tropical escape, or the simple freshness of a garden delight, it's all about teasing—and pleasing your palate. To titillate my taste buds, I always reach for cayenne pepper. The spice adds that extra zing to my blends, and its' warmth and energy are like a sassy salsa party. Try it! Sprinkle some sass into your own concoctions.

Let's Get Tropical – *frosty, fabulous, almost a piña colada*
- ¾ cup coconut water
- ½ medium banana, sliced into chunks
- ¼ cup pineapple (fresh is best), diced
- ¼ cup cauliflower, diced or rice
- ½ cup plain Greek or nondairy yogurt
- 1 tsp. coconut oil
- 3 mint leaves
- Shredded or flaked coconut as a topper

Spicy Date Shake – *creamy, dreamy, and deliciously exotic*
- ¾ cup almond milk (or milk of choice)
- 1 small banana, sliced into chunks
- ¼ cup sweet potato, peeled and cooked
- 1 serving of vanilla protein powder
- 1 tbsp. chia seeds
- 1 Medjool date, pitted and torn into pieces
- Cinnamon and cardamom spice (don't stop till you get enough!)
- Dash of cayenne pepper
- Crushed pistachios as a topper

Zen Goddess – *clean, green, a refreshing touch of enlightenment*
- ½ cup 100-percent orange juice (freshly squeezed is best)
- 1 kiwi, cut into chunks
- ¾ cup cucumber, cut into chunks
- ½ cup silken tofu
- ¼ cup avocado
- Cilantro - go wild!
- 1 tbsp. orange zest as a topper

Smoothie Packs

When I know I have a super-busy week ahead, I set aside a small block of time to make my own convenient, customized smoothie packs, so I have a wholesome meal ready to go at a moment's notice.

Making these little kits in advance elevates the whole experience, from prepping a single smoothie to throwing together a smoothie party for the week! Just stock your freezer with pre-measured packs, and whenever you need a smoothie, simply toss the frozen contents of a bag into the blender with your liquid of choice—and voila! Blitz away. Once you get into the routine of prepping, you will feel like a boss each morning, and you'll thank yourself for being prepared and having a healthy meal close at hand.

Through trial and error, I have learned a few tricks to ensure a smooth kitchen experience.

- Use ingredients that are easy to source, in season, and that can be mixed and matched in various ways.
- If you use frozen fruit, purchase those with no added sugar.
- Chilled liquid is best; alternatively, you can add a couple of ice cubes to give a creamy texture.
- Tweak your smoothie's texture. If you want it smoother, toss in some extra liquid or choose lighter fruits and veggies. In the mood for something thick and delightful, add less liquid, turn it into a smoothie bowl, and enjoy it with a spoon.
- When using whey or plant-based protein powders, make sure it is the purest form possible, without added chemicals and artificial sweeteners.
- It's totally Zen to substitute ingredients with similar alternatives, so be daring—try new combinations of foods and listen to your palette.

Arrive, anchor, and unearth your energy.

Summarize your intention for launching your smoothie-making practice.

....

....

- List the produce and equipment you will need.
  ....
  ....

- What tweaks does your ritual need?
  ....
  ....

- What are you learning about yourself through this practice?
  ....
  ....

Be your own smoothie queen and power up your morning, one sip at a time. I am forever grateful to Mr. Smoothie King, who, in trusting in the nutritional power of the smoothie, paved the way for the drink we all know and love today. By trusting *your* precious self, you can spark your self-love revolution, and it can be as simple as starting with this daily nutrient-dense ritual. Remember why you're doing this: to feel good, to be energized, and to keep your mojo in check.

SOAK YOUR INNER SELF
Sassy Sips for Perfect Hydration

Naked
or gussied up,
sparkling or still. Natural
or naughty. Icy, tepid, or steamy hot.
Shower yourself from
within, one sacred
drop at a
time.

Random camel fact: Did you know that camels can survive for weeks without drinking water, and when they finally do, they can drink the equivalent of three and a half kegs of beer within three minutes?! Another fact: Humans are not camels. And nor should they ever try to be.

Some time ago, I had the pleasure of partaking in a camel safari through the Thar desert in India. The lovely Lala, a flirtatious, eye-fluttering camel, would be my fun ride as I gracefully lurched across the desert for two hot, unhurried days. As we set off, several large bottles of icy water dangled from Lala's saddle; they were my water supply until we returned to our Indian oasis.

As we ventured over the rolling dunes and zigzagged through the scarce vegetation, the relentless sun bore down on us, transforming our water bottles into little ovens. Not fancying drinking boiling water in the desert (at least without a shot or two of coffee), I embraced my inner camel and willfully waited it out. Perched upon Lala for two days, I hee-hawed and hallucinated, taking only sips of what was absolutely necessary to avoid landing myself in an Indian infirmary.

Silly girl.

Boy, was I as stubborn as a mule—or a camel in this desert-water-crisis case. Fortunately, this story had a happy ending. Returning from safari, I was presented with a gloriously icy three-liter bottle of what was arguably the most delicious water I had ever tasted.

Dare I ask if you've ever felt as excited as I was over the mere act of drinking cold, clear water? Not really? Water consumption can present some curious questions if we think about it. How much should you consume each day, and how can you ensure you get enough? What if you don't love the taste of plain old water? How can you tell if you're dehydrated, and what's water got to do with mojo anyway? So many questions, so little water! Sweet reader, I suggest you pour yourself a large glass of aqua and settle in.

Despite being odorless, colorless, and tasteless, water is a nutrient critical to our health and vitality. Without it, we would literally shrivel up and die. Our bodies are made up of over 60 percent water, and retaining ideal levels of moisture throughout the body, including our skin, is partly due to sufficient water intake. Drinking water helps to lubricate, protect, and cushion our joints, spinal cord, and tissues.

You know that feeling when your eyes, nose, or mouth becomes dry? This is a sign you're dehydrated. Research shows that we tend to 'dry out' as we age—yikes! So if your outsides look as parched or as crusty as the soil in the Thar desert, it could be a sign that your insides aren't happy either.

Could you agree that your water bottle is like a dear friend you enjoy hanging out with or more like an annoying aunt whom you only tolerate in small, infrequent doses? Throughout our day, we may forget to stay sufficiently hydrated; we get busy, and it's hard enough to remember what's on our to-do list, let alone to drink up, especially if we're not feeling parched.

No big deal, or Achilles heel? Did you know that brain fog—that fuzzy-headed feeling that can creep in unexpectedly—is often associated with dehydration? Lack of fluids can affect our mental clarity, mood, and ability to get a succulent night's sleep—all mojo-worthy factors that allow us to live our sweet little lives to the fullest!

Our clever body needs to eliminate toxins to function properly, and it does this through sweating, peeing, and pooping. Replenishing the water lost through these natural functions assists our kidneys with doing their job of filtering out the nasties. We can keep hydration balanced by ensuring more fluid goes into us than out. As for how much water do we need? Most research agrees—it's wise to start with half your weight in fluid ounces. So, for a 130-pound woman, that's 65 fluid ounces—eight glasses (8 fl oz./240 ml) of refreshing hydration every day. But remember, we're all unique, so pay attention to your body's thirst cues, as each individual has specific requirements. If you're an active go-getter, living at higher altitudes, in a warm climate, or managing a health condition, consider adding an extra glass to stay refreshed.

Inch Inside. Ponder your current drinking habits.

What is the first thing you drink when you wake up? How does this make you feel?

....

How much water do you roughly drink in a day? Glasses, ounces, or milliliters.

....

✏️ *Do you often feel dehydrated?*
....

A simple baseline test is checking the color of your urine. The lighter your urine, the greater the chance you are well-hydrated.

Follow the Flow. Yes, we need to follow the flow! Pun intended! Let's do the math.

✏️ *Calculate how much water you should be drinking using the following formula. To convert your weight from kilograms to pounds, multiply your figure by 2.2. Take your weight in pounds, halve this, and you have your daily water intake in fluid ounces.*

....

Now that you know the importance of staying hydrated and have an idea of how much you should aim to drink daily, let's dive into how to create a simple yet life-giving ritual for your mornings. This ritual will make sure both your cup of water—and your mojo—runneth over!

The Joyful Toolbox

We often start with the best intentions, but staying on top of our hydration game can be challenging in the hustle and bustle of life. To tackle this, I prep my daily water allowance in advance, taking the guesswork out of the equation. By creating a water station first thing in the morning, I'm showing some love to my body right from the get-go. A practical visual cue can keep us on the right path. Try these two easy tricks to keep you sipping throughout your day.

If you are based in one location and can easily access a pitcher or bottle from a central place in your line of vision, then what I call *pitcher perfect* might be a swimmingly good option. Each morning simply fill your container with fresh water and pour from it throughout the day. I like to use a brightly colored large drinking bottle with measurements displayed, making for easy tracking.

If you are out and about or travel for work, you may prefer *bottles to go*. Fill several plastic bottles—I like to use BPA-free and pop them into an insulated carry bag, ready for your day. You can take what's needed as you go about your business. When I began using this strategy, I found it helpful to number each bottle to see how I progressed throughout the day. At night I rinse the empty bottles and get them lined up, ready to refill the following morning. To give you an idea, I fill five sixteen-fluid-once (500 ml) bottles, which total my daily quota; the number of bottles you fill will depend on how much they hold and your daily water intake. Whatever strategy you use, the goal is to have your daily water quota inside *you* (and not the container) by the time you go to sleep.

Decorated Water

If drinking plain water isn't your jam, you must decorate it—truly! It's delicious! Citrus slices, cucumber, berries, watermelon, and a variety of spices, such as ginger, are just a few ways you can add a little va-va-voom to your naked H_2O. Blending these ingredients takes only minutes, tastes incredibly refreshing, and is natural and chemical-free. Experiment with the ingredients you have on hand and change the quantities to make a larger or smaller batch, or to suit your taste. There are no rules, so do what tastes good to you! On a side note: you will want to prepare these blends well in advance to let the water become sufficiently infused. I make a batch the night before and store it in the refrigerator, so my water station is deliciously primed to go the following morning.

The following recipes each make approximately sixty-four fluid ounces of infused water. Preparation is easy. Firstly, wash and cut up the produce you want to infuse, place it at the bottom of a bottle, jar, or pitcher and fill it to the top with clean, cold water. Once infused, you may prefer to strain the water to remove the produce. An alternate method is to make smaller batches in a cocktail shaker and strain as you go. Here are some recipes to get you started.

Minty Cucumber Lime
- ½ small cucumber, sliced
- 3 slices of fresh lime
- a small handful of fresh mint leaves

Orange Vanilla Cinnamon
- ½ orange, sliced
- ¼ tsp. pure vanilla extract
- 1 cinnamon stick, broken into pieces

Minty Citrus Ginger
- ½ lemon, sliced
- 3 tsp. grated fresh ginger
- a small handful of fresh mint leaves

Blueberry Vanilla Lime
- ½ cup fresh or frozen blueberries
- 1 fresh lime, sliced
- ¼ tsp. pure vanilla extract

Strawberry Mojito
- ½ cup fresh or frozen strawberries
- 1 fresh lime, sliced
- a small handful of fresh mint leaves

Still on the fence about getting your daily aqua quota in? Try these hacks. They work, and they're fun.

Try adding a dash of *cayenne pepper* to add some pizzazz to a drink. Research has shown that spice, especially capsaicin, boosts the body's ability to break down fat and burn more energy, thus revving up the body's fat-burning processes. And the spiciness can make you feel thirstier, which is a great way to get drinking!

A deceptively effective strategy is to *change the temperature of the water*. Start your day with warm water to wake you up gently, and if you *sip through a straw*, it will make you consume more water and faster too. For those desiring to lose weight for health reasons, *drinking a small glass of water before each meal* can help you feel fuller and not overeat. If you're still unsure how to make your habit stick *post small stickies with reminders to drink up* wherever you keep snacks or set *notifications on your smartphone* for intervals throughout the day until your new habit is routine.

A Handbook for Sparking a Sassy Morning

Arrive, anchor, and unearth your energy.

🖋 *Summarize your intention for launching your hydration practice.*

....
....

🖋 *List the materials and resources you will need.*

....
....

🖋 *What tweaks does your ritual need?*

....
....

🖋 *What are you learning about yourself through this practice?*

....
....

What is your body telling you today about how you can up-level your self-care? In what ways can you shower yourself more from within? Whatever your preference is—icy, tepid, sparkling, or still, it's possible to make the healthy habit of staying quenched fun. Establishing the morning ritual of preparing a daily water station takes you one step closer to living with mojo, which is feeling more refreshed, energized, and alive every day. Go now and shower yourself with love, sweet reader!

Heart

GLOW WITH GRATITUDE
Awaken Your Awe and Count Your Blessings

Sunshine
*through the window.
The smell of freshly brewed coffee.
Hearing the right song at the right moment.
That first oaky, buttery sip of chardonnay.
A magic wand called mascara.
Gel pens and a fresh page.
Christmas in April.
Nana naps.
AirPods.*

It is a classic car clog. As we crawl past a charming Catholic church, I can't help but think this is immaculate congestion. After all, traffic inching forward at a painfully relaxed pace, bumper-to-bumper, is part of livin' la vida loca in Mexico. I switch off the fresh air supply from the Jeep's dashboard, and chemical exhaust fumes from neighboring space invaders gradually fade.

My mood fluctuates between mild irritation and sheer exasperation when the car behind us starts honking. Every other vehicle in the jam follows suit and begins to do the same. Do they think this will bring them closer to divine car-cluster-free intervention? A match ignites in my belly.

It fuels the fire within me, bringing to the surface a tantrum about to be unleashed. I sit with it for a moment, exhaling slowly. Then, somewhere deep down, I hear that small voice of reason nudging me.

Stop for one hot second, Lisa. You know what you need to do. It's time to play the Grownups' Gratitude Game.

You will learn how to play this game in the Joyful Toolbox section.

Think back to yesterday. Was it a *good vibes* day? Perhaps the sun was positively shining, and you slayed your to-do list, squeezed in a coffee date, and nailed that icky meeting with enough energy left to power up a small island. You climbed into bed feeling all virtuous and complete, *filled to the brim with gratitude*. Oh, joy! Or maybe you weren't vibing at all? Gratitude eluded you, and the day was as frustrating as eating a hamburger with freshly painted nails. Just not gonna happen, is it?

Of course, showing gratitude is easier when life is blooming roses. Your mojo is high, and you feel gracious even toward the garbage truck that crawls noisily past your bedroom window on your Saturday morning sleep-in. But what about when things aren't going well? What if we don't feel like being all Pollyanna-like? After all, gratitude isn't supposed to be a platitude, a solution, or a promise we must keep, right?

Finding a wee moment of awe can be tricky when the clutch of negativity squeezes the life out of you. Days when you feel like crap and wonder when the next pudding will turn to poop (an expression from Somebody's Granny on the internet, which I just love) make gratitude challenging. Even when a thorny moment presents itself, like being in the middle of a Mexican traffic standoff, it can drown out our graciousness. But that's where the sweet spot is, sweet reader—among the rubble of our messy moments.

If we hit the pause button for just one nanosecond and tune into ourselves we're already showing some self-love. Whether we flip a sticky situation with positivity or take a moment to hold unexpected blessings, gratitude can light up our day and bring fresh purpose and joy.

In Melody Beattie's book *The Language of Letting Go,* she defines gratitude as "turning what we have into enough and more." Moments of gratitude needn't be big. They could be small, fragile, and awesome. By adding up all the tiny wonders in our life right now, there's a sense of fulfillment, however brief, which can elevate even the most squashed mojo.

> **Inch Inside.** When was the last time something so delicious happened—a time when you wished you could bottle up the magic and keep it forever?
>
> *Set a timer for one minute, and brainstorm what you are grateful for in your life right now, at this moment. It could be specific people, random surprises, small moments, or particular possessions. Whatever you choose, be as explicit as possible.*
>
> ....
> ....
> ....
> ....
> ....
> ....

> **Follow the Flow.** While setbacks can affect our happiness factors, try this exercise.
>
> ✒ *Write down a small challenge you have in your life at the moment.*
> ....
> ....

Now flip it over and reframe it. What tiny lesson are you learning about yourself? Find the small silver lining, a teeny light at the end of the tunnel, or just a pocket-sized positive thought you are grateful for through that challenge. Write it into the frame below.

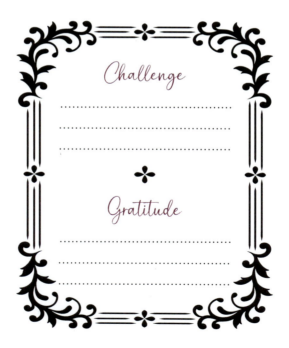

The Joyful Toolbox

I dare you to play the *Grownups' Gratitude Game*. Try it solo, or with other exasperated humans, big or small, as a distraction to lift your mood and unfunk yourself. Take the first letter of your name and identify something you are thankful for that starts with that letter. Brainstorm as many things as possible—and get creative when you run out of the obvious! For example, Liesa is grateful for lollies (that's Kiwi-speak for candy) and for *like-minded ladies who love lattes and lacy leggings*. You get my drift. It can get quite ridiculous, which makes it even more fun—and effective.

Optimism is like a key to unlocking our inner joy, no matter the situation we're in. This tiny game of gratitude? It's my recipe for a joyful occasion, every time. With each playful thought, I'm whisked away to a world of more positivity, completely absorbed in the present moment.

I've also made it a habit to *give thanks for one thing each day before I even get out of bed*. Every little blessing sets the stage for a more vibrant and mindful day. It's the perfect way to start my morning, and it sets the tone for a day filled with positivity and purpose, boosting my mojo and overall well-being.

Creating a memorable daily ritual that can take gratitude to the next level while keeping us anchored in the present moment is something I treasure every day. You can establish a practice that fosters gentle accountability and consistency by keeping a record of gratitude, which can help you start and stay in your day in a purposeful way.

Over the years, I have used various forms of visual "gratitude-minding," enabling me to record thanks in unique and meaningful ways. Here are four different methods that may resonate with you.

My all-time favorite is the *Good Vibes Jar*, a rather beautiful way to recall those moments. Simply cut up fifty-two small pieces of colored paper—yes, one for every week of the year, although you can prepare these weekly too. Place the papers into a large jar, and at the end of each week, write a few statements of gratitude on a piece of paper with the date, and then pop it back into the jar. Continue this practice every week, or if you prefer, take it up a notch and write a gratitude note each day instead of weekly. The more you express gratitude, the brighter your days will become.

I recommend showcasing your jar in a prominent spot, like by your bed or in your office, as a daily reminder to give thanks. As the year struts to an end, I gleefully cozy up with a glass of wine to dive into my treasure trove of gratitude goodies. It's a heartwarming and joy-filled way to wrap up the year!

If you love pretty things, like me, you may wish to decorate the vessel that holds your gratitude notes with favorite colors, themes, and materials. Decorating the Good Vibes Jar is a perfect primer to begin your practice; it's a noteworthy act of self-love, and you will already have a note of gratitude to pop inside when you've finished your wee work of art.

Then there's the *Noble Notebook*. This method is an easy way to record thanks in one portable place. Each morning I list two or three things I am grateful for or, depending on my mood, sometimes I fill a whole page in the notebook with one particular marvelous moment. My notebook is small enough to fit easily into my bag, ready to record on the go.

Find a new notepad from around the house, or, if you prefer, there are a vast selection of blank notebooks you can buy, as well as some with prompts and days set out, ready at your fingertips, if you prefer a more structured approach. I often open a notebook page randomly to read past entries on less-than-stellar days. It always brings a smile to my face to know that despite how I'm feeling at that moment, there is always something to be grateful for. That simple act of reflecting, even for a short moment, is enough to turn your attitude into gratitude.

If you're a visual person or just like having a daily reminder posted around your office on colorful Post-it notes, you may find inspiration in the *Stickies Strategy*. Source a pad of Post-it notes—they come in a rainbow of colors and shapes these days, and distribute them around your house or workspace. I keep a small stack by my bedside, in my office, and even by my coffee maker, anywhere I might feel inspired to record a thankful moment. As inspiration strikes, I'll grab a stickie and write a note of thanks throughout the day. But I don't stop there. I like to post gratitude around the house! I adorn the bathroom mirror, inside my diary, bedside lamp, or my significant other's coffee mug. Not only is this an act of loving-kindness towards myself, but it also keeps me in the present while brightening up someone else's day.

If you know your heart is full of gratitude, but your mind draws a blank, nab this *Grab Bag* strategy. Each day choose one of the following questions to focus on. If you're like me and thrive on an element of anticipation, simply copy each sentence onto small separate pieces of paper and put them into a small container, or even the Good Vibes Jar, and randomly select one each day.

- What is something you've learned this week that you're grateful for?
- How is your life more positive today than it was a year ago?
- What is your favorite part of your daily routine?
- What makes you beautiful?
- Describe a recent time when you truly felt at peace.
- What is a hard thing you've recently done that led to personal growth?
- Describe your favorite moment of the day.
- What is a small win you've accomplished in the past twenty-four hours?
- Tell of a time when you laughed out loud this week.

Arrive, anchor, and unearth your energy.

🔖 Summarize your intention for launching your gratitude practice.

....
....

🔖 List the materials and resources you will need.

....
....

🔖 What tweaks does your ritual need?

....
....

🔖 What are you learning about yourself through this practice?

....
....

Eckhart Tolle, spiritual teacher and self-help author, mindfully states: 'Acknowledging the good that you already have in your life is the foundation for all abundance.' So, take a second to amuse yourself with the *Grownups' Gratitude Game*, give thanks for a small blessing as your feet hit the floor each morning, or start your daily practice using some of the ideas above. When we embrace the wonder in every moment, we don't need to wait for a 'special moment' to ignite it. You light your day with possibility, curiosity, and joy when you flick the gratitude switch. So go ahead, sprinkle some gratitude, sweet reader—that's the magical power of gratitude and embracing your mojo!

SHAMELESS SELF-LOVE
Brush Up Your Senses One Stroke at a Time

Lavish
those curves,
find comfort in your own skin.
Embark on the voyage of a delicious caress,
a moment of daily dalliance
to renew and awaken
and bask in this
moment.

It was 1987. I was scrubbed within an inch of my poor, dear life. Picture this: an opulent, gleaming, domed marble room with tall ceilings, stained-glass skylights, and walls adorned with gorgeous mosaics. I had stumbled upon a traditional Turkish bathhouse, *a Hammam*, tucked away in the enchanting alleys of Old Istanbul. This was way before the whole Hammam craze took over, and there I was, a wide-eyed backpacker, eager to experience the sacred cleansing ritual of having my body, soul, and maybe even my brain, washed. I'm sure I needed it all!

Stepping into the bathhouse was quite the experience. My eyes scrutinized the scene with uncertainty as I gripped the humble cloth that I was gifted a little more tightly around my body. Through the steamy haze, I spotted a burly figure charging my way: none other than my spa attendant, the fiery *natir,* Fatma. With a flick of her hand, she directed me to lie on the marble bench, and in a flash, that tiny towel was whisked away, leaving me with my racing thoughts and naked body. Let the adventure begin!

What followed was an hour of excruciating bliss. The bathing ritual alternated between being showered with hot water and brushed and burnished with a *kese*, a Turkish exfoliating cloth. It was unexpected. It was shameless. I was rubbed raw. Every inch of my body was on fire. It was only the following day that I noticed how soft, exfoliated, and glowing my skin felt. Those clever *natirs* were on to something.

Hot springs, saunas, steam rooms, and hot baths: there is something truly gratifying about surrendering to the bliss of a good soak or relaxing in a heated room. It delights the senses and satisfies the soul. Add a massage or body scrub (or a swift scouring in a Turkish bathhouse), and you might just have the perfect mojo-worthy spa-dulgence experience.

Ancient bathing rituals have paved the way for an array of body-care and well-being practices that have developed into the spa culture we know today. Your lovely spa therapist can scrub, knead, or massage your woes away, along with untying that annoying knot in your neck. It's a chance to bliss out in the moment *and* reap the benefits post-treatment—it's a skin-win situation.

Our body is an incredible work of construction and art. Did you know that your skin—the body's largest organ—wraps around twenty square feet on your fabulous frame? That's another reason to love the skin you're in and take good care of it. Cold climates, scorching heat, dry air, indoor heating, hormones, sun damage, food imbalances, and toxicity (phew!) all play a part in the quality of that precious real estate.

When I was just seventeen, I was told by an insightful woman that up until age twenty, we have the skin we are born with, and after that, we have the skin we deserve. It meant little to me at the time. After all, this freckly-faced teen still had *three years* to go till I needed to even *care* about how dark that statement could be. My aha moment appeared when that wise woman's words came back to bite me on the bum, or should I say my nose, around age forty—as I was having yet *another* benign but worrisome mole removed from my face. Sweet reader, please wear sunscreen every day and protect your skin. Let's practice some self-love in action.

Inch Inside. Sit down with yourself and take a deep breath.
If your body could talk right now, what would it say to you?

....
....

Follow the Flow. Allow your mind to recognize each amazing thing your body allows you to do each day.
Using the letters of your first name, write a positive word or statement about your body next to each one.

....
....
....
....
....
....
....

Now read aloud the words from the previous exercise, thanking your body for each attribute as you go. Imagine it as a love note to your body.

A girl can dream of spa days to zap life's stress away. But who's got the time and cash for that daily treat? I've created my home-spa-adise—and it's open all day, every day. In my PJs, it's my little escape—waving goodbye to stress from head to toe, releasing tension for both my mind and body.

Whether we like it or not, as we grow older, our skin becomes less efficient at detoxing and naturally shedding dead skin cells. Changes such as roughness, loss of elasticity, dryness, and thinning can become a reality long before we're mentally ready. However, it's never too late to honor yourself and start a body-care routine that will help preserve your skin for decades. I take pleasure in a daily body-care ritual that puts self-love into action. It only takes a few minutes and offers me a moment to connect with my physical self. It leaves my skin tingling and glowing—every day. And it's not what you might think . . .

We brush our hair and teeth, and even cleanse and polish our faces with a brush. But have you ever considered the idea of extending "the brush of love" to the rest of your body? Ancient Egyptians were pioneers of dry brushing, using natural enzymes like sour milk and wine for exfoliation, unveiling their soft, supple skin. This age-old dry body brushing technique remains relevant today, offering a beautiful way to invigorate your skin and bathe it in gratitude. And the best part? No milk needs to be spoiled or wine uncorked (unless you're in the mood for a celebration while you soak).

Dry body brushing combines exfoliation and massage by using a dry brush to perform short, firm strokes over your body. How is this ritual worth your time and energy? Read on, sweet reader.

This invigorating ritual enhances blood circulation to your skin, providing an amazing tingle that will get your blood pumping. Before getting dressed, embrace the power of dry brushing, as it can truly be a game-changer for your energy levels. Have you ever felt sluggish or lethargic? Research shows that it could be your body's way of saying, "Hey, my lymphatic system needs some help!" Dry brushing to the rescue! When done regularly, this body-loving practice can unclog and stimulate your lymphatic system, clearing away toxins and stress that can otherwise drag you down.

And then there's exfoliation. Who doesn't love a good shedding of the past? Whether that's releasing bad energy or sloughing old skin, dry brushing removes grime and oil, and dead skin cells, resulting in increased cell turnover and skin that is left smoother and more radiant. The bristles of the brush manually sweep away dull, rough, flaky skin cells, improving the appearance. No need for messy scrubs! After a dry brushing session, your skin will feel softer and ready for greater absorption of body-care treatments immediately afterward.

For me, a core benefit of dry brushing is that it really is an act of self-love. When you dry brush, you are taking care of every inch of your body; it's a moment to reconnect with what is truly yours and to appreciate all the incredible things your body does for you. I also use my brushing time to check my skin for pesky moles, lumps, or bumps that often go unnoticed. I can't recommend this enough.

The Joyful Toolbox

The very cool thing about dry brushing is you don't need much to get started—just a good-quality brush. Most dry brush experts recommend those with natural bristles which are made from plant sources like jute, sisal, and even cactus fibers. Natural fibers are softer and less harsh on the skin. Brushes come with or without a handle: a long handle enables you to reach your back and other awkward places, but I prefer a handheld brush which is easy to maneuver over everywhere else. These can be easily sourced at online stores, pharmacies, department stores, or health shops, so check out a few styles to see what appeals to you.

Dry brushing is a breeze, and with a little practice, you'll find right technique for you. Start by shedding those layers and embracing your birthday suit. (Go on—check your incredible bod out in the mirror as you do so!) Grab your trusty brush and begin from the feet, sweeping upwards along your legs with smooth, flowing strokes. Give some love to those tricky areas behind your knees and move upwards, caressing your inner thighs, stomach, breasts, tush, and if you can manage it, your back too. Don't forget your arms. Start at your hands and work your way up to the shoulders, using gentle yet firm strokes. Adjust the pressure as needed—go easy on delicate skin and apply more force where needed, like the tough soles of your feet. Oh, and trust me, don't dry brush if you have SUNBURN—ouch! Remember, dry brushing should be a soothing experience. If it feels uncomfortable, you might be brushing too vigorously. Take it easy and let the brush do its magic. Afterward, if you shower, give your skin some extra love with moisturizer to seal in all your hard work. To keep your trusty brush in tip-top shape, give it a gentle shampoo bath at least twice a month. This will bid farewell to any dead skin buildup and keep it ready for many more blissful dry brushing sessions.

Arrive, anchor, and unearth your energy.

🖌 *Summarize your intention for launching your body brushing practice.*
....
....

🖌 *Note your preference for a body brush.*
....
....

🖌 *What tweaks does your ritual need?*
....
....

🖌 *What are you learning about yourself through this practice?*
....
....

Historically we have been led to believe that self-indulgence is a sin, but how can the upkeep of that fabulous body of yours be anything less than a delightful duty of care? Indulge your mojo through the small yet mighty ritual of dry brushing and use it as a loving way to connect with your body with each sensual stroke. Sweet reader, be the goddess you are, and give your skin the gorgeous glow it deserves.

Spirit

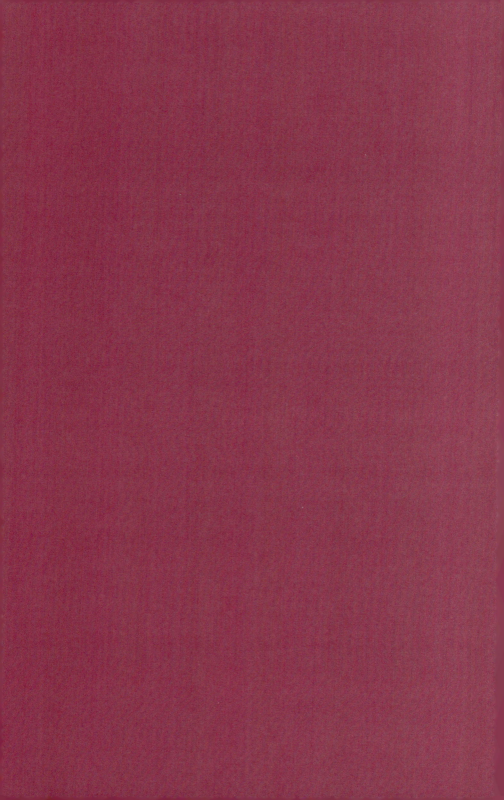

MS. MEDITATION MAVEN
Breathe In and Let It Flow

Clouds
*of consciousness
drift past me, some heave—
about to burst into inky chaos. Others
glide past in lightness of being—wispy, luminous,
and delicious. They journey through
the landscape of my mind
as I float between
the spaces.*

Feeling a little crispy, a little fried, I nervously raised my eyes toward the surgeon and mustered the courage to ask, "But how did this happen?"

After an emergency medical evacuation to Singapore to remove a chunk of gangrene the size of a golf ball from my stomach, the doctor's words struck me like lightning. "You reached the operating table just in time. Sepsis had started to manifest." Bug-eyed and bewildered, I could only stare in disbelief. How naïve of me to think that my fit and healthy lifestyle would shield me from unexpected calamities of the urgent medicinal kind.

During my lengthy recovery, questions still haunted me. Amidst the doctor's orders of mandatory rest and medication, I decided to venture into something new. "From Burned Out to Refreshed," the title of a daily meditation on my newly installed app, sounded delightful and just what my frazzled brain and broken body needed. It marked my first encounter with *guided meditation*.

Setting the stage, a cozy, extra-warm LED light basked with anticipation under my Bali umbrella lampshade. In the quiet corner of my office, I eagerly anticipated the stillness and silence of the early morning. With headphones in place, I settled onto my yoga mat, tapped the play arrow on my smartphone, and closed my eyes. I was ready for it all.

However, distractions crept in—my nose itched, thoughts of a nasty email I had just sent flooded my mind with guilt, and my left foot fell asleep as a neighbor's dog relentlessly barked. How on earth was I going to do this?

Calling upon the cosmic Zen masters, I took a long, slow, deep breath in, surrendering to the velvet voice of the meditation maestro. Whatever woo-woo was going to happen, I was determined to stay present. It was only six minutes long after all.

Admittedly, it took some practice. It's hard to be still! Maybe you relate to this too. During my meditation experience, I was absurdly antsy, despite it being only a few minutes long. I felt a little foolish as if I were being watched and judged by an invisible force, and my mind was still racing from the unanswered questions I had collected since my health scare. But as I embraced meditation as part of recovery, my body started to heal, my mind began to crack open, and I learned to give myself some grace—one breath at a time.

Since introducing meditation into my lifestyle, I flow more gently. Whatever obstacles present themselves throughout my day, meditating, especially in the morning, means I feel more grounded and better equipped to tackle them. It's been a large part of regaining my mojo.

I have literally learned to breathe again.

A Handbook for Sparking a Sassy Morning

Did you know that our breath—an anchor to the present moment, accessible to us at all times—can coax us into stillness? Through meditation, conscious breathing slows our heart rate and allows our mind and body to synchronize, bringing us more into the present moment through sensation. This lets us calm our racing minds by learning to observe our incoming thoughts, *whatever they are,* and accept them without needing to change or action them. There's no judgment of right or wrong, as every thought, feeling, and emotion is valid as part of the human experience.

Maybe you're familiar with the "monkey mind." You're anxious and overwhelmed, with a million thoughts rushing through your head. This unwelcome visitor sabotages and undermines our ability to think clearly *every time.* Scientists estimate that humans have around 70,000 thoughts per day, and a worried or anxious mind can generate a new negative thought every few seconds. Yikes!

When my monkey mind begins to spit and howl, I lovingly tell her I know she's there before returning to my breath. "Oh, hi, Overwhelm; I see you've come to visit. Take a seat." *Return to the breath.* "Excitement, you've arrived! We will celebrate another time." *Return to the breath.* "Pissed-offed-ness, ooh, look at you. Over there, please." *Return to the breath.*

Approaching my incoming thoughts in a direct, yet gentle and compassionate way, helps me remove any judgment toward them while keeping me anchored in the moment. It's empowering to learn that acknowledging a thought but not engaging in conversation can lead to focused calm. And that keeps the monkey at bay.

Raise your eyebrows if you meditate, but is it more for an emergency than a regular ritual? This used to be me. I'd stop and start meditating like I was a fifteen-year-old learning to drive a stick shift. Turning to meditation in a tough spot (as I illustrate in the Joyful Toolbox section of this chapter) can bring a much-needed sense of calm, but often, that's where it ends—easily forgotten as the moment slips away. It's like sticking on a Band-Aid— a quick fix, covering the wound just for now, and then tossing it aside once things heal up, not giving it a second thought until the next problem pops up. Shifting my approach, I worked meditation into my morning routine. Starting each day with it means I'm better prepared to face challenges. And when life gets rough, I've developed a more effective way to handle it.

Sweet reader, let yourself on your morning voyage through meditation with these exercises.

Inch inside. Think of a quality you yearn for more of each day— love, balance, peace, belonging, joy, laughter, vitality, etc. Use this intention to write a positive affirmation.

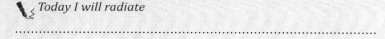 *Today I will radiate*

....

Follow the Flow. Use your intention to settle into this simple breathwork exercise below.
First, read the meditation to familiarize yourself and then follow its guidelines as you take a few moments to BE in the present moment. Follow the sensation of your breath as it goes in and out. Notice when your mind has wandered by acknowledging the thought, then return your attention to the breath.

> *Be kind to yourself.* Don't obsess over the content of your thoughts as they arise. Welcome them all. Just return to your breath.
>
> *Find a quiet spot,*
> *relax your body and*
> *close your eyes. Rest your shoulders.*
> *Put your hand on your belly and take a long, slow, deep breath*
> *—in through your nose. Hold it at the top for three counts,*
> *then release it through your mouth*
> *as you make an audible sigh.*
> *Repeat, and this time as you breathe in, mentally say, "I am."*
> *As you release your breath state your intention.*
>
> **What did you notice? Did you feel your breath?**

I love the simplicity of this mindfulness meditation. It can be used anytime, anywhere, and it's a quick and effective way to center, re-energize, or iron out some of the wrinkles of life that are causing you stress throughout the day. It helps bring awareness of what you're sensing and feeling in the moment without interpretation or judgment. Space is created where you can pay attention to your thoughts by simply observing whatever arises and using breathwork to gradually let them be. It's a beautiful act of self-love as we get *to feel it all* and bring some softness back into our world.

The Joyful Toolbox

Choosing a meditation style that fits can feel like trying to find the perfect pair of comfy yoga pants—so many choices, but you want the one that hugs just right.

If the mindfulness meditation above resonated with you, consider revisiting it as a focal point to connect with your breath. And remember my tale of my first encounter with guided meditation? Still today, this method continues to light my fire and fill me up.

Guided meditation is like a friendly hand to hold on to during your mindfulness journey—no prior experience needed! It's an effective practice that anyone can try and embrace. The best part is that you'll have a teacher or facilitator guiding you through the whole experience, using their voice to help you relax, center, and focus. It's like having your own personal mindfulness guru. With such a wide range of topics, teachers, and techniques to explore, there's something for everyone in the world of guided meditation. And the best part? You can easily access this vast resource base online or in person, making it super convenient to dive into this calming practice.

Before I invested in a meditation app, I used videos from the internet to explore the kinds of meditations that vibed with me. There are hundreds of meditation channels on YouTube, many of which can be accessed for free. With a bit of surfing, you can find something suited to your particular preferences, needs, and timeframe.

With the abundant choices of available meditation apps, you can access hundreds of meditation sessions and programs at your fingertips. Each one offers diverse topics and themes, such as managing anxiety and stress, work and productivity, breathwork, happiness and positivity, sound healing, soothe and heal, self-care, and travel. There are also meditations for specific challenges, such as parenting struggles, grief, body image, test prep, recovery, pregnancy, healthy eating and exercise, and handling chronic pain. Of course, this list is incomplete; if you can think of an emotion or a particular challenge, there's sure to be a guided meditation.

I am a late bloomer with technology-based *anything*, yet when I began practicing guided meditation this way, it helped me stay in the present moment with just the swipe or a press of a finger. It was practical, met my needs, and it was convenient. No matter if you're home or away, with minimal scrolling, you can participate in pre-recorded or live video or audio sessions, and even book a private session with an expert if you choose to.

I use digital calm not only as part of my daily morning practice but also throughout the day, especially if it's become a little prickly.

I was still in my comfy jammies as I took out the trash early one morning when, to my horror, I accidentally pulled the house security gate shut, inadvertently locking it behind me. A brief wave of panic coursed through my body as my mind started spinning with the logistical nightmare before me. I was holding a trash bag and my smartphone, but there were no keys. I glanced around at the quiet neighborhood street, feeling a little like a trapped raccoon.

With my heart racing, I clutched the device in my hand, a desperate thought swirling in my mind. After a few quick calls to arrange an Uber and retrieve a spare key from hubby's workplace, I opened the meditation app on my phone. As I perched on the street curb, awaiting my ride, I took a deep breath, closed my eyes, and tuned into a soothing guided meditation. In the midst of the morning bustle, I found a moment of peace and calm.

As the soothing voice in my ear guided me through my moment of panic, I felt the tension in my body slowly ease away. The anxious thoughts subsided, and I started to focus on the present moment—the chirping birds, the gentle breeze, and the soft touch of the morning sun on my skin. It was like I had found a moment of serenity amidst the chaos of my predicament. As the Uber pulled up, I couldn't help but feel a wave of unexpected serenity washing over me. Stepping out in my cozy J.Crew PJs, I thanked the amused driver. A little unconventional? Maybe. But that's the magic of finding calm wherever you are.

Whether you prefer to do a self-directed or guided meditation, you only need a quiet place to practice. For the latter, headphones or earbuds can enhance the experience, but they aren't necessary. Create your own special ambiance with soft lighting and a favorite aroma. I like using my essential oils diffuser, which I discuss in the chapter on "scentual" awareness.

Before you begin your meditation, get yourself situated: lie on a yoga mat, sit in a chair with your feet on the floor, sit on the floor or a mat loosely cross-legged, or you can kneel. There's no "right way" to do it; just make sure you are comfortable and can maintain your position for the length of the meditation.

Arrive, anchor, and unearth your energy.

Summarize your intention for launching your meditation practice.

....
....

List the materials and resources you will need: device, access to the platform of choice, mat, candle, stool, etc., and think about when and where you will set aside time to meditate.

....
....

✒ *What tweaks does your ritual need?*
....
....

✒ *What are you learning about yourself through this practice?*
....
....

When we incorporate meditation into our mornings, we give ourselves the best opportunity to become fully aware, fully awake, and fully alive. It allows us to gently launch our day instead of our day launching us. If practiced consistently, meditation allows us to be grounded in the present, to sit with our thoughts, warts and all, and *let them be.* And, while we may be legendary human-doings, nothing beats living this life with mojo—as a joyful human BEing.

"SCENTUAL" AWARENESS
Get in the Mood in a Whiff

Rich,
freshly brewed
coffee wafting out from the
open doors of a nearby espresso bar
transporting you back to a tiny
café in Rome where you
visited years ago.
Bellissimo!

It is a sultry summer's night as I joyfully make my way through Hyde Park toward an evening of beautiful music beneath the stars. The rest of the world around churns in the background—the click of heels, the babble of voices, and the collective energy splashing against the canvas of London's arresting architecture. I'm lost in a moment of pure anticipation of a glorious night of musical romance. Quickening my pace, I unexpectedly sense the familiar. My nostrils flare, I stop in my tracks, and my heart skips a beat. A welcoming whiff of *Obsession* wafts through the air and draws me to my past.

BOOM! It is 1986. A boyfriend with a permed mullet (a less-than-savory but oh-so-popular hairdo back in the day), a totally radical graduation night, and dancing to the DJ's beat of Whitney Houston's "How Will

I Know" overwhelms the senses. This night was the night my rolled-up slouch socks fell out of the teeny strapless bra of my ball dress and flung across the floor like meatballs.

Oh, I remember.

The night of mullets and meatballs was undoubtedly a moment of déjà vu I did not expect, but, oh, the vivid memories it stirred up! Can you recall when the whiff of an aroma hurled you back into a timeless vortex? Who was there with you at that moment? How did it make you feel? What emotions surface when you take in that scent now? My obsession with *Obsession* could raise a lot of questions.

The power of scent, also known as olfaction, occurs when a smell is directed through your olfactory bulb, the region in your brain closely connected to your amygdala and hippocampus that manage memory and emotion. Scientists know that smell can affect work performance, behavior, and mood. So, what drives our behavior can be affected by the scents we surround ourselves with. To me, smell is the most mysterious and fascinating of our five senses. It can spark a memory, transport us to another time and place, or change or create a certain mood—all within a whiff in a nanosecond.

Back in my days of teaching kindergarten on the island of Bali, I had an unexpected and heartwarming encounter with nostalgia while setting up a student activity station with Play-Doh—the colorful molding clay we all know and love. As I held that squishy dough under my nose, my past collided with the present in the sweetest way, lifting my spirits in an instant! The scent of Play-Doh brought me back to the carefree weekends I spent with my sister, Claire, when we were little. We'd elaborately craft teacups and bickies (the Kiwi version of cookies) for our dolls and stuffed animals. Those were the days of pure joy and fearlessness, and Play-Doh played a magical role in bringing back those cherished memories. I was so taken by the moment of remembering that I even carried a little ball of dough with me for days afterward.

I passionately associate scents with mojo, which is why I enjoy incorporating "scentual" awareness into my daily routine. Taking a few minutes each morning to set up what I fondly call a "scent station" is self-love in action. It's where my senses can flirt with me, playfully luring to the surface my needs and desires for the day ahead. By choosing the right "scentual" mood elevators, we can transform our energy, improve our mood, and become a more badass version of ourselves. That's mojolicious!

Aromatherapy and Essential Oils
My day begins one drop at a time using essential oils' natural and healing properties. While these oils have been used in wellness practices for thousands of years across numerous cultures, more recently, they have gained worldwide recognition as more people discover alternative health treatments and age-old remedies for feeling good. Welcome to aromatherapy, the practice of using essential oils to promote well-being and (I might add) a feeling of fabulousness!

Essential oils are, in essence, plant extracts. They are made by steaming or pressing various plant parts (flowers, bark, leaves, roots, seeds, nuts, or fruit) to capture the compounds that produce fragrance. Their healing qualities begin when they are inhaled or applied to the skin.

Inch Inside . . . to the past. Think of a time when scent played an important part in a particular moment or memory.

✎ *Describe the incident in vivid detail if you can.*

....
....
....
....
....

Follow the Flow . . . to the present. We all have aromas that we associate with happy, positive vibes.

✎ *Once you have read the Joyful Toolbox, list some aromas and methods of "scentual" awareness from this chapter you would like to try.*

....
....
....
....
....

The Joyful Toolbox

If you're curious about how to incorporate essential oils into your morning routine, in this box of tricks, you'll find some *scents*ational ways of doing so. We'll focus on six essential oils I use most often; each is versatile, easily sourced, affordable—and, when blended—produce a range of mood-enhancing qualities. They smell absolutely amazing. Of course, you can also experiment with other essential oils. Find which resonates with you.

Before we start, I have to give the disclaimers. *First, regardless of the blend or oils you use, if there are any signs of skin irritation or headache, stop using the oil immediately and never administer oils to inflamed or broken skin. Second, I am not a healthcare professional, and the information in this chapter is based on personal experience and research, and is for general informational purposes only.*

Six Superwomen Oils
Lavender is my number-one go-to essential oil. It can calm nerves, balance emotions, help with sleep, and promote well-being.

Orange is another feel-good-factor oil that is uplifting to the body and mind. It also fosters creativity and supports a positive mood.

Peppermint wins my vote for increased alertness and concentration while invigorating the senses. I use it to energize before a workout or focus when I have a pesky assignment due.

The gorgeous floral scent of *ylang-ylang* is both calming and relaxing. It feels like a tropical trip in a bottle, reminding me of my travels to the spice island of Zanzibar.

Lemon promotes vitality as it excites the senses and enhances mood. It is also remarkable for cleansing negative energy.

And finally, there's *warm and spicy ginger* that stimulates and soothes. It inspires positivity and promotes and balanced mindset. Best of all, ginger feels like being wrapped in a cozy fleece blanket.

So, you may ask, how should I use these wonderfully versatile essential oils?

I use *Palm Inhalation* for a quick pick-me-up throughout the day. Dab a drop or two of essential oil directly from the bottle onto your palm. Rub your hands together vigorously, and then, cupping your hands over your nose, slowly breathe in the aroma. The oil dissipates rapidly, so this technique is particularly effective when you want an immediate mood shift. I use this oil inhalation before a workout, if I feel a stressful situation coming on, or if I need some inspiration before settling into a project. It's a quick and effective way to help me stay in my day.

First thing each morning, I set up my *diffuser*, so within minutes my office is filled with a gorgeous scent. In aromatherapy, an oil diffuser is a device that breaks essential oils down into smaller molecules, dispersing them into the air for an uplifting or calming effect, depending on the oil that's being used. Being free of chemicals, I prefer them to freshen a room than using commercial room sprays. Add 100ml (about 3 oz) of water to the diffuser, up to seven drops of your essential oils of choice or follow your diffusers' instructions and experiment with your amounts. Then switch on your device and let your senses be lifted. You can find diffusers at health shops, grocery outlets, department stores, and online stores.

Practicing *Kitchen Aromatherapy* with a few supplies from your garden or kitchen is an alternative way to use essential oils. I like to keep fresh herbs such as lavender, cilantro, rosemary, and mint handy as they release a wonderful scent once rubbed between your fingers. Fresh citrus peel can be potent and function as a wonderful mood pick-me-up, whereas fresh lavender has wonderful soothing qualities. Pop a sprig or two of lavender into a small glass container, cover it with olive oil, and leave it to marinate. After a few days, I use it as a nourishing hand moisturizer when it has released its scent. If you don't have access to a diffuser, you can create your own simply by simmering one or two cinnamon sticks in a small pot on the stove, letting the aroma waft throughout your kitchen.

Blends to Create the Mood

When choosing the mood you seek, let your nose guide you. It's fun to experiment and find your signature blends. Here are some of my favorite mood-elevator combos to get you started. Each essential oil is shown in drops as measurements. Find what you're feeling and get blending!

If you feel your *confidence* is missing in action: 3 lemon, 2 peppermint, 2 orange.

Need to be *uplifted* and get out of that funk? 3 lavender, 2 ylang-ylang, 2 peppermint.

Perhaps it's time to snuggle into that blanket of warmth and *comfort*: 3 ginger, 3 orange, 1 ylang-ylang.

Get into the zone and increase *productivity*: 3 lemon, 3 orange, 2 ylang-ylang.

Power up and *energize*: 3 lemon, 2 lavender, 2 peppermint.

Mental *clarity* is a priority: 4 lemon, 3 ginger.

Finding quality oils takes a little homework, as standards for quality control of essential oils don't currently exist in the United States. Reputable companies use the formal Latin name to identify the plant ingredient and the extraction process used to produce the essential oil. These are good places to start. There are many brands and price points to choose from, and they are easily sourced online as well as in supermarkets, health stores, and specialty shops. Finding a quality oil that feels right for you is worth it.

Arrive, anchor, and unearth your energy

🌶 *Summarize your intention for launching your "scentual" awareness practice.*

....
....

🌶 *List the materials and resources you will need.*

....
....

🌶 *What tweaks does your ritual need?*

....
....

🌶 *What are you learning about yourself through this practice?*

....
....

Using essential oils can be a gentle and loving gift to yourself. Whether you want to recreate a moment or upgrade your mood, incorporating oils into your everyday self-care practice will help you move throughout your day with mojo. And you're only a whiff away, sweet reader.

Meltdowns, Mindset, and Mojo

"Bloom where you are planted" was the promise blazoned across my Mexican-themed flowering cactus storyboard that I had just finished constructing. I'd recently relocated to vibrant and colorful Mexico City, and there were exciting challenges ahead: a new country to explore, a different language to learn, another tribe of wonder women to seek, and fresh goals to aspire to. I felt energized, optimistic, and ridiculously joyful—my mojo was in full bloom!

Except, several weeks later, the world went deathly quiet, and conversations, consciousness, and countries started closing down. The only thing in full bloom was my sense of impending uncertainty. Routines felt labored, and mornings were lethargic. Feeling completely isolated in unfamiliar terrain, I could have surrendered to the "I-don't-give-a-shit-anymore" mindset as my confidence teetered on taking a one-way ticket to Hasta-la-vista-ville. I felt blooming awful.

What about when the shit hits the fan, and the universe screws up? What happens to mojo then?

Life has a knack for serving up poop pudding, but as I've discovered, taking a break and starting fresh helps to avoid getting a bad taste in your mouth. I was caught in my morning funk, realizing my morning routine had lost its sparkle, so I connected the dots. The toolbox of insights and wisdom was right at my fingertips, and my inner Goddess was ready to blaze a trail. 'Take a breather, honey, rally your spirits, change it up, but don't you dare lose that spark!' she told me. (I like sparkles—I wasn't about to risk it.)

Rewriting the script, adjusting the rules, shaking things up . . . sweet reader, take the next, small step that feels right for you.

A Handbook for Sparking a Sassy Morning

In the midst of my Mexican meltdown, I turned to my bag of tricks and adjusted my morning routine to keep me centered. Instead of longer meditations in my office followed by a full-on workout, I opted for three-minute meditations while lying in bed, followed by the *Wake Up Between the Sheets* routine. I prepared smoothie packs in advance, so I knew I had a healthy meal at my fingertips when I didn't have the energy to make one. I was amazed by my emergency-multitasking skills of prioritizing a daily walk to release stress as I journaled into my smartphone while finding little things to be grateful for along the way. Three rituals in one! These were simple tweaks but were just what was needed to keep the spark alive in my mojo. I was paying attention to the self-care I needed at that moment.

Diving into the four pillars of wellness—mind, body, heart, and spirit—felt like finding a well of energy and happiness that kept me going throughout the day. Over time, my morning routine became a part of me, way more than just a habit. These rituals launch my day, making a special moment in the quiet of dawn when my mind's at its sharpest and the day's loaded with potential. You, too, sweet reader, can design a morning practice that's as customizable as your Spotify playlist, setting the mood for a day that's all about you. Turn your daily habits into your personal morning party—because who doesn't love some self-love shenanigans?

Living MoJOYfully

As you've discovered within the pages of this book, the four cornerstones of well-being are the keys to creating a nurturing and enduring morning routine. Focus on these as you design your personal rituals, infusing your mornings with purpose, positivity, and renewed energy.

BODY: *Prioritize your morning "iTime."*
Allocate it on your calendar, and be intentional about your physical well-being and the tasks you need to accomplish. Research suggests that when you write down your intentions and allocate time for them, you're 42 percent more likely to follow through.

HEART: *Celebrate your ritual.*
Find the sacred in your rituals, make it a ceremony, and create something unique that deeply resonates with you. This personal connection infuses each day with a special spark. Creating your vibe is your superpower!

MIND: *Review regularly.*
Once a week, take time to reflect. Add, tweak, or remove anything that no longer serves you. You and your morning practice are a continuous work in progress, so embrace imperfection and nurture your mental well-being's growth.

SPIRIT: *Go gently.*
These rituals are designed to reduce stress in your day, not add to it. Start with one, give it time to grow, and when you've established its place in your morning, introduce another, and so on if you choose. Just as the rituals nourish your spirit, remember to adjust your morning practice to align with the ebbs and flows of your life.

As we wrap up this book, you might be thinking, "I should have it all together by now. I've just devoured a whole self-help guide; surely my mornings will be nothing less than a coffee-fueled fairytale!" It's a lovely thought, sweet reader, but life's twists and turns have a way of keeping things interesting. There will still be moments of discomfort, times when joy seems distant and snarly moments when you just want to curl up or unleash your frustrations into a pillow.

Here's the deal: Self-care is about celebrating YOU; it's about finding what clicks for YOU. It's about nurturing the parts that make YOU gorgeous: your mind, body, heart, and spirit. And it all begins with rituals—your rituals. So go ahead, fashion your mornings in your own style. Prioritize yourself, and you'll discover the heart of self-care, where living with that inner spark becomes your new superpower. And you know what? No one, absolutely no one, can mess with that!

MoJOYfully Yours,

Liesa xx

About the Author

As a wellness mojo-ologist and devoted transformation coach, Liesa's passion is to seize life and decorate it her way. What exactly is a mojo-ologist? Imagine having a wingwoman to help you unveil your most vibrant 'mojo'—that special spark within, and infuse moments of joy and occasion throughout your day.

With a diverse background as an international educator, certified personal trainer, nutrition specialist, and group fitness instructor, Liesa brings a dynamic blend of expertise, skills, and a dash of sass to her work. She has passionately guided and empowered countless women worldwide, helping them craft their personal haven of shameless self-care.

Inspired by the challenges and triumphs on her quest for well-being, Liesa penned the book *Don't Mess With My Mojo* after perfecting the morning faff—otherwise known as the frustrating art of fussing, flapping, and failed attempts that left her feeling anything but fabulous. Overly underwhelmed and unproductively over it, she decided to push back and reclaim her mornings.

Drawing from personal experience and savvy understandings, readers are led through the stages of creating mornings that brim with curiosity, freshness, and fun—so there are fewer other irritating f-bombs and way more mojo! Her debut book reveals the secrets behind her treasured yet sassy way of embracing this wild and precious life, inviting readers into a world of genuine joy and vitality.

A globe-trotting Kiwi ex-pat, Liesa understands the significance of ditching the "should-ology" and diving into YOUR-ology—except when presented with a delightful glass of oaky chardonnay.

Sweet Words of Praise

"You've landed, and that's exactly how I felt reading this book. Liesa's distinctive brand of humor and raw honesty lovingly coaxes the reader on a joyful jaunt to mojo."

—**RACHEL SUERY, MEdPsyc.,**
Psychologist | Wellness Coach | Consultant at www.suerycoaching.com

"A true passion project that is aimed to give us the chance to know ourselves better, to find that spark that will reignite our souls, and to help us soar to our highest potential. A book to keep close by."

—**MAAN GABRIEL,**
Author of *After Perfect* and *Twelve Hours in Manhattan*

"Packed with personal anecdotes and self-exposure, this book resonates, making you realize it's also your story. Unlike typical well-being books, it doesn't dictate what you must do. Instead, it prompts self-reflection, encouraging simple changes for lasting benefits to mind, body, and soul."

—**HELEN MORSCHEL, M.Ed.,**
International Education Consultant | Health advocate